Track Your Plaque

Track Your Plaque

The *only* heart disease prevention program that shows you how to use the new *heart scans* to *detect, track, and control* coronary plaque

William R. Davis, MD, FACC
Foreword by John Rumberger, PhD, MD, FACC

iUniverse, Inc.
New York   Lincoln   Shanghai

Track Your Plaque

iUniverse, Inc.

For information address:
iUniverse, Inc.
2021 Pine Lake Road, Suite 100
Lincoln, NE 68512
www.iuniverse.com

The information contained in this book is not intended to represent a medical diagnosis, treatment or medical advice in any way, as it is general information and cannot be relied on without consultation with your physician. It is not intended nor is it implied to be a substitute for profession medical advice. In fact, taking full advantage of the Track Your Plaque program will *require* that you consult with your physician, or a physician willing to work with you. As medical information and your health can change rapidly, we strongly encourage you to discuss all health matters and concerns with your physician before beginning new diagnostic or treatment strategies.

ISBN: 0-595-31664-6

Printed in the United States of America

Contents

Foreword ix

Introduction vii

Chapter 1   Track Your Plaque 1
             Why diagnosing silent heart disease is still a roll of the dice.

Chapter 2   Your life is worth $60,853 18
             Hospitals are in the business of heart disease.
             You are in the business of prevention.

Chapter 3   What your doctor didn't tell you about heart disease 26
             Why measuring coronary plaque is the most important
             health test you can get.

Step 1

Chapter 4   Heart disease can be measured 43
             A "yardstick" for coronary plaque

Chapter 5   Want to know whether you have heart disease?
             ...Know your score! 56
             Everything you need to know about heart scanning

Chapter 6   Can I reduce my heart scan score? 70
             If we can accurately measure coronary plaque,
             we should aim to reduce it.

Step 2

Chapter 7   "My doctor said my cholesterol was fine...
             So why did I have a heart attack?!" 77
             Why cholesterol fails in so many people

Step 3

Chapter 8   LDL cholesterol and beyond: The many causes of
             heart disease and their treatments 87
             How lipoproteins make the causes of coronary plaque
             seem obvious

Chapter 9   The six Track Your Plaque nutrition principles 108
               Eat right to gain control of your plaque.

Chapter 10   Control your plaque with exercise and weight-loss 137
               Slash your need for medication and supercharge your
               program with these tips.

Chapter 11   Use nutritional supplements to control plaque 156
               Choose the right supplements to add real power to your
               program.

Chapter 12   Track Your Plaque Personal Profiles 172
               Stories of real people in the Track Your Plaque program

Chapter 13   Putting together your own personal
               Track Your Plaque program 185
               Follow the 3 easy steps for control of your plaque

Appendix A   A Review of the Scientific Evidence 193
               The Use of Calcium "Scoring" as a Surrogate Marker for
               Coronary Artery Disease

Appendix B   How to find a heart scanner in your area 209

Appendix C   How to arrange lipoprotein testing in your area 237

Appendix D   Resources to help you find tools
               and products used in **Track Your Plaque** 241

Index 247

Acknowledgements

Preventive cardiology is experiencing a technological boom. But these new tools are leading us into uncharted territory in heart disease prevention. In assembling the crucial pieces of the Track Your Plaque program, there was no textbook to read, no guidelines to lean back on, no single expert to consult. The concepts in this book therefore reflect the product of many people's contributions.

I've long been an admirer of Dr. John Rumberger, among the few world's experts in heart scanning. Dr. Rumberger first introduced me to heart scanning several years ago. I will be forever grateful for his gracious generosity in devoting many hours to imparting much of his knowledge and experience. Dr. Rumberger is truly a visionary who has doggedly pursued projects always with the goal of getting at the truth. Looking back at his original work of over 15 years ago, I am still in awe of his clinical foresight.

Closer to home in Milwaukee, I owe many thanks to the dauntless work and persistence of Steve and Nancy Burlingame, who provided the financial know-how to erect the first heart scanner in Wisconsin. The staff at Milwaukee Heart Scan, likewise, have helped carry the torch of this concept in our region. This tough, smart group has succeeded in a town that often resists change.

Of course, no amount of thanks can make up for the behind-the-scenes dedication that my wife, Dawn, has provided. She sacrificed many nights and weekends to allow me to pursue this project, but her enthusiasm was unflagging. My love, always.

On the eve of the completion of this book, Dr. David King passed away. Dr. King, physicist and originator of many of the basic concepts of heart scanning, will be missed by many in the heart scanning community as a gentleman and educator, and among the few who possessed the foresight to comprehend the power of this technology.

Foreword

U.S. healthcare is an immense $1.65 trillion dollar system that boasts some of the finest, most advanced technology available in the world. The American Heart Association estimates that societal costs for cardiovascular care in 2004 alone will grow to $368.4 billion. Nevertheless, the number one killer of men and women, coronary heart disease, still continues to flourish. Why is that? Are we getting any closer to a truly effective solution?

Not quite. Lost in the flurry of technological advancement is heart disease *prevention*. This poor relation of high-tech cardiovascular care suffers from lack of attention—but, in my view, it is the key to our healthy futures as individuals, more than any high-tech procedure. My research efforts over the past 25 years have, therefore, focused on the concept that heart disease can be detected early, before it causes symptoms, while it may still be a controllable process.

Dr. Doug Boyd and colleagues from the University of California San Francisco put their heads together over 25 years ago in his modest tinkerer's laboratory, where he had conceived a means to circumvent the limitations of the slow scan speed of conventional CT devices. The device developed was (and still is) an engineering marvel, but it lacked practicality for heart imaging. Several years later, working with Dr. Boyd, we meshed my research on imaging of the heart and the composition of coronary plaque, managing to bring clinical cardiology to the world of CT imaging to begin to answer the question of whether coronary plaque could be easily measured in patients with Dr. Boyd's "ultra-fast" imaging technology.

Thus, a whole new approach to early heart disease detection was born. First, some background:

It is a fact of basic biology that the presence and amount of calcium detected in a coronary artery by a CT heart scan accurately reflects the presence and amount of atherosclerotic plaque build-up. Calcium can form in plaque *years* before the development of symptoms, such as chest pain and shortness of breath.

The new CT heart scanners are precision tools that allow us to accurately measure, down to a millimeter, the quantity of calcium in your plaque. This permits us to calculate a calcium "score". A calcium score is computed for each of your coronary arteries based upon the volume and density of the calcium.

Your total coronary calcium score obtained using electron beam CT or some of the faster, more recent multi-detector CT systems is a precise and validated measurement of calcified plaque and a very good estimate of total plaque burden. Numerous studies have confirmed that the coronary calcium score is highly predictive of a future heart event.

Other imaging tests (echocardiography, nuclear stress testing, MRI) are incapable of measuring heart plaque burden. For instance, tests like stress testing are only abnormal when there is already a blocked artery or very advanced heart disease, but don't measure plaque in your heart. Cholesterol testing does not see or measure heart disease. In fact, the total cholesterol values of people who do and who don't have a heart attack are about the same!

The causes of plaque build-up are many and include age, sex, genetics, environment, lifestyle choices, smoking, cholesterol values, levels of blood pressure, obesity, and diabetes, to just name a few. The problem is that the result of all of these factors on your coronary risk is impossible to determine just by physical examination and standard blood tests. The heart scan looks at *you,* and the results reflect *the sum total of all of these factors* over the preceding years. Thus, in terms of predicting risk, it is better to look at *you* as a unique individual, rather than looking at you as a statistic related to your current cholesterol value or other indirect measures of risk.

If you have plaque, the best way to reduce your risk of heart attack is to retard or stop further plaque build-up. Studies have shown that people who slow or even stop plaque growth substantially reduce their risk of heart attack. Your physician has many options to help you accomplish this, including reducing risk factors, quitting smoking, diet, exercise, vitamins, cholesterol lowering medications, and diabetes and blood pressure medications. Since you now have a baseline score, you have the ability to measure whether your heart disease has stabilized or even regressed. That is, you can **Track Your Plaque**! It is very important that you work with your doctor to stabilize plaque disease, but the biggest factor in this equation is *you.*

A major issue in taking charge of your life is to make the decision with your doctor to get a baseline heart scan. The next step is to understand what the results mean and how you can effect regression or at least stabilization of the plaque volume. The difficulty is that often there is no resource for the education that allows you to "put it all together"—until now.

Dr. Davis is one of those rare cardiologists who "gets it" with respect to primary prevention of heart disease. He has put together in **Track Your Plaque** a wealth of clinical information condensed for the average patient to understand, but complete enough to become a handbook for the seasoned clinician. Read this book, underline sections, make notes in the margins—this is *the* single resource that can help you fully grasp the *power of prevention* now possible with our exciting, new technologies.

John A. Rumberger, PhD, MD, FACC
Clinical Professor of Medicine, The Ohio State University, Columbus, Ohio
Medical Director, HealthWISE Wellness Diagnostic Center, Dublin, Ohio

Introduction

May, 1995. I exited the room of an intensive care unit patient, an accountant, who'd just survived his second heart attack and was awaiting bypass surgery. He was among several patients I'd seen that day with heart attacks, heart failure, and recovering from major heart procedures. My pager beeped as I entered the nursing station. I froze mid-step when I saw the number beginning with 201— the area code of my hometown in New Jersey. The cold fear of family crisis gripped me. I grabbed the nearest phone and hurriedly dialed the number. It was picked up on the first ring by my sister, June. She got straight to the point. "Bill, Mom died last night."

I was stunned. "How did it happen?" I asked. She told me that a friend had discovered Mom's body, cold and dead from a heart attack while in her sleep. She was 62.

How could this be? I'd spoken to my mother just days before and she'd been feeling fine. She said nothing about pain in her chest, breathlessness, nervous feelings—nothing. She was active, ate well, and had seen her doctor just two weeks earlier.

It took a few minutes for me to collect myself and face the situation. But it took several weeks for the irony of my mother's death to sink in. Here I was, a busy interventional cardiologist, performing balloon angioplasty, inserting stents, carving plaque out of patients' coronary arteries, yet my own mother had died suddenly of a disease I thought I knew how to treat.

This personal tragedy sparked a life-changing realization for me: What I did professionally as a cardiologist was fundamentally and terribly flawed. It shattered my long held belief that I was delivering the best care to my patients. Years of training and practice, doing the same as thousands of my colleagues, but it took my mother's death to help me begin to see how misguided the conventional approach to heart disease really was.

I began to see that my colleagues and I tackled heart disease as "crisis management." We waited for a crisis like heart attack, then proceeded to "fix" it. Every day was an exercise in triage, tending to the sickest people first, relegating the less sick to a lower priority. We focused on catastrophes, pulling patients back from the brink of tragedy, but devoting little thought to why they were there in the first place.

I came to understand that, despite the apparent success of crisis management, attempts to identify people with heart attack in their future are *wrong 90% of the time*. Yes, you could make statistical predictions by looking at cholesterol, but too many of us have seen people with normal cholesterols succumb to heart disease. We've also seen people pass stress tests only to die of heart attack weeks later. The sad fact is that *the overwhelming majority of heart disease comes as a complete surprise to both victim and doctor*.

It's well established that coronary heart disease is a process that begins in childhood, silently lurks and grows over decades until finally declaring itself with a heart attack, resulting in death in half its victims. If 50% of men and 35% of women die this way, that means that silent heart disease is everywhere, yet its potential victims proceed through life entirely unaware.*

Through my frustration, I wanted answers to several questions: 1) How can coronary heart disease and risk for heart attack be identified *years* before catastrophe strikes, 2) How can this risk be reduced or eliminated with greater certainty than provided by crude measures like cholesterol, and 3) How do we measure and *prove* success?

After several years of effort, I believe that a rational, effective program is now available. I call it **Track Your Plaque**. Once you understand these concepts, I believe you will agree that the answers to these questions are really maddeningly simple. In fact, you may find that the answers to many of *your* questions about heart disease have been available all along, but you just didn't know where to look. You may also be angered by the misguided beliefs of people around you—perhaps including your doctor—who insist that heart attack is not a predictable event, or that it is inevitable, or that the only effective treatments are hospital procedures. It's all untrue.

For many people, the concepts we will discuss may change the course of their lives. A path of silent heart disease that eventually manifests as catastrophe can be changed to another of control over coronary plaque over a lifetime. What began as a tragedy for me has led to a life of health for my patients and myself, unmarred by the scars of the cardiovascular hospital system. As the family member of a victim of heart disease, as an "insider" in the cardiovascular healthcare system, and as a fellow human being hoping to see people around me avoid an all-too-common fate, I hope to convey these same ideas to you.

---

* In this book the phrase "heart disease" will, for simplicity, mean coronary heart disease, and does not include valvular heart disease, conditions of heart muscle (cardiomyopathies), pericardial diseases, and other systemic disorders that affect the heart.

Chapter 1

Track Your Plaque

Why diagnosing silent heart disease is still a roll of the dice.

"Doctor, will I have a heart attack?"

You walk into your family doctor's office. Your neighbor, exactly your age, just died from a heart attack—no warning, good health beforehand. In fact, you chatted with him just days before while he took a break from push-mowing his half acre lawn. He looked fine. Understandably shaken, you want to know whether you have silent heart disease though you, too, feel fine. You really press the doctor for an answer. How does he/she answer your question? More than likely, it would go something like this:

1) "Do you have chest pains or excessive breathlessness?" he/she begins. You respond that you have no symptoms.

2) An examination follows. Everything is normal, with no physical sign of heart disease.

3) You get an EKG. The doctor declares that you've not had a heart attack.

4) Your doctor checks your cholesterol values. Your total cholesterol and LDL cholesterol are average, neither terribly high nor low, or perhaps they're moderately elevated.

5) A stress test is performed. It's completely normal.

You leave the office with advice on cutting the saturated fat in your diet and plans to have the cholesterol tests repeated in several months. After the entire process, you'd probably be satisfied with your doctor's thoroughness. You're convinced that you have no hidden heart disease and won't fill the cemetery plot next to your neighbor.

1

Think again. *Nothing* that your doctor did detects hidden heart disease. You could have extensive silent heart disease or you might have none. You could drop over dead watching your favorite reality TV show next week or you might outlive all your neighbors until your 95th birthday. For the great majority of us, none of these tests distinguish these two drastically different fates. All your doctor managed to do was look for extremes: a very high cholesterol value, heart disease symptoms, a severe reduction in heart blood flow by stress testing.

The reality is that *90% of future heart attacks will not be detectable by any of the above tests.* The vast majority of doctors would follow the sequence of testing described above, not much different than taking a roll of the dice with the odds heavily stacked against you. All too frequently, false reassurances are provided that hidden heart disease is not present. Rely on the conventional approach, and you're very likely to lose this gamble.

Clark's story is an all too common example:

Clark is a 45-year-old research chemist at a pharmaceutical company. Clark and his wife, Angela, experienced dramatic changes in their lives when they recognized that one of their children was mentally disabled. Now eight years old, their disabled child's special needs seemed a full-time job between transporting to school, counselors, and doctors, not to mention the constant attention required at home. Living in a community that provided the quality of education and counseling that Clark and Angela wanted for their child was a priority, but resulted in an hour-long commute each way to Clark's work.

Despite their extraordinary stress, Clark maintained a hopeful and grateful attitude for his family's lives. Perhaps this caused him to simply dismiss the fatigue he began to suffer at age 39. He thought it was just the stress of his unique family demands. Several visits to his doctor resulted in much testing but no diagnosis. Despite an EKG, stress test, and laboratory work, no mention was made of any heart-related issues. His doctor, in fact, praised Clark on his favorable cholesterol levels.

A chance conversation with a colleague at work prompted Clark to undergo a heart scan. The result: Clark had an extreme amount of plaque in his coronary arteries, so much that his arteries appeared solid "casts" of calcified plaque. Further investigation led to a heart catheterization that disclosed one coronary artery completely closed and the two others hanging on by a thread, resulting in a coronary bypass operation several days later.

Clark's heart scan probably saved his life. Imagine if he had undergone this test five years earlier. Perhaps, if he and his doctor had recognized his critical heart disease at age 40, Clark could have been spared the pain and hardship of bypass surgery. That's what **Track Your Plaque** can show you.

The new age in heart disease detection

Add to Clark's story the hundreds of thousands of similar tales that unfold every year in this country, many ending in tragedy. Much of this tragedy and human suffering is simply unnecessary. Armed with the knowledge and technology already available, you can avoid these painfully common fates for you and your family.

The development that will crush the current crisis management approach is the availability of imaging technology that allows detection of hidden coronary plaque. Where cholesterol testing, stress tests, and other outdated methods of identifying heart disease have failed us, the new methods of silent plaque imaging hold tremendous promise. You and I now have access to tools that were only dreamt of 10 years ago.

Over the last decade, there has been an explosion of technology permitting easy and accurate detection of *silent* coronary plaque. While the world focuses on cholesterol and high-tech hospital care, thousands upon thousands of research studies have been completed validating the power in detection of coronary plaque. The rapidly accumulating data show that knowing and *quantifying* the amount of plaque you have is *the most powerful predictor of future heart attack available.*

If you smoke…

If you smoke, stop reading this book right now and consider returning it to the bookstore for your refund. Let's make this clear right from the start: If you smoke, nothing can substantially reduce your risk for heart disease unless you quit. In other words, even if you did everything else right, the adverse effects of smoking so overwhelm all positive influences that you will fail. If you smoke, just plan on your heart attack…or stroke, lung cancer, throat cancer, gastric cancer, abdominal aneurysm, emphysema, loss of your feet or legs from poor circulation.

There are many resources that can help you quit smoking. One good place to start is your physician, who has several strategies that are widely available. Your pharmacist can also help, as can many organizations like the local branch of the American Lung Association that offers lectures and support groups. Of course, no program, no matter how good, will help unless you truly want to quit.

Like Clark, it is not uncommon for people with low cholesterol values and no symptoms to have hidden coronary plaque uncovered by these new technologies. Conversely, there are many people who live in daily fear of succumbing to a heart attack because of a family history of heart disease, or high cholesterol, only to find out that they have absolutely no coronary plaque and therefore nearly zero risk of heart attack in the near future. The concept of heart scanning can shed light on all these situations.

What is Track Your Plaque?

Track Your Plaque is your information resource on how to apply this new approach. You won't have to wait for life-threatening symptoms, nor rely on cholesterol numbers. You won't have to depend on some intuitive feeling that you might have a heart attack. Tracking your plaque tells you whether you have coronary plaque, how much, and what the future holds. It is a real world method of managing heart disease risk that anybody can follow.

Track Your Plaque can show you, in three basic steps, how to identify and then seize control of heart disease in your life. In Step 1 of this proven approach, you'll be shown how to detect hidden coronary heart disease, even years before danger strikes. The most widely available method to detect silent heart disease is coronary calcium "scoring" obtained through the increasingly available electron-beam or multi-detector heart scanners. Direct measurement of hidden coronary plaque eliminates the murkiness of "risk factors" like cholesterol testing, and the unacceptable imprecision of stress testing. These new technologies make the identification and precise measurement of coronary plaque a safe, inexpensive, 10 minute process that just about anybody can obtain.

In Step 2, you'll be shown how your heart disease is (or might be) caused with the powerful technique of lipoprotein analysis. This exciting technology easily pinpoints the causes of heart disease even when cholesterol testing fails. Time and again, people who've survived heart attacks are told that no cause for their heart disease could be found. Yet when lipoproteins are tested, the causes seem almost obvious. Greater insight into the causes for heart disease arms you with powerful tools to control coronary plaque.

Once your coronary plaque is scored (Step 1), and its causes pinpointed through lipoprotein testing (Step 2), you can then begin Step 3, applying effective therapies that can, with proper guidance, reduce or eliminate the prospect of heart attack or major cardiac procedures in your lifetime.

Track Your Plaque is therefore a three-step program that shows you how to:

1) Detect and measure coronary plaque

2) Identify the causes of your coronary disease

3) Effectively treat the causes in order to arrest or reduce the amount of plaque you have.

Track Your Plaque is *not...*

Have you seen the books that try to wow you with descriptions of high-tech procedures like transplantation and artificial hearts? **Track Your Plaque** is *not* another book that helps you comprehend the world of cardiac medicine so that you enjoy a measure of comfort as you are led like lambs to the slaughter.

Track Your Plaque is also *not* a new diet that, by eliminating or adding certain foods, boasts of a "cure" for heart disease. Let's face it: eating more broccoli or less red meat will not "cure" heart disease. Nutrition is important, but no matter how good your diet, it does not cure the genetic causes of heart disease. It is only a part of the final answer. In fact, you can *double or triple the quantity of coronary plaque* in your arteries in a year's time while feeling fine, eating a low-fat or low-carbohydrate diet, or following an extreme fitness program. Precisely measure plaque, and you can gauge with confidence whether disease has progressed or not. As coronary plaque grows, the danger of heart attack and death grow with it. Conversely, as coronary plaque shrinks, so does risk of heart attack and death.

A brief history in coronary plaque detection

Why are you hearing about this earth shatteringly different approach to heart disease now? Why couldn't we do this 10 years ago?

In past, detection of silent coronary plaque was impossible except through autopsy or hospital procedures like heart catheterization. You'd therefore have to suffer a catastrophe and die or have a major coronary event like heart attack to have plaque detected.

Several technologies have been developed that make detection of silent plaque a widespread reality. Along with these technologies, scientific and clinical understanding of the causes of plaque growth has boomed. These combined developments now allow us to assemble the necessary pieces of a program that can, for many of us, "shut-off" coronary plaque. These technological milestones include:

1983   *Physicist Douglas Boyd, PhD develops electron-beam technology that permits extremely rapid CT scanning at speeds sufficient to image the moving human heart. CT x-ray beams are rapidly focused by electromagnetic fields rather than mechanical motion of the scan device.*

1985–1995   *Contrary to prevailing opinion, several clinical studies demonstrate that* mild *coronary blockages (e.g., 30–40%) are far more likely to cause heart attack than severe blockages (e.g., 90%).*

1988	Drs. Ronald Krauss and Melissa Austin of University of California-Berkeley publish their research that connects lipoprotein disorders with risk for heart attack.
1991	Dr. James Otvos, a physicist, applies nuclear magnetic resonance imaging (NMR) to measure and characterize lipoproteins in human plasma, making lipoprotein measurement inexpensive, fast, and highly accurate.
1995	Dr. John Rumberger of the Mayo Clinic proves that coronary calcium can be used to measure total coronary plaque volume. He validates this measure using Dr. Boyd's EBT scanner, demonstrating that the quantity of plaque can be accurately measured using this device.
1998	Drs. Traci Callister and Paolo Raggi of Vanderbilt University describe the use of coronary calcium "scoring" as a means of tracking growth of plaque and document numerous cases of plaque shrinkage.
1998–present	Clinical evidence accumulates showing that coronary plaque can be tracked, arrested, and often reduced.

You can see that the technology of scoring coronary plaque is hardly a decade old. But in that brief time, a critical mass in technology and understanding has been reached and the field has exploded. You and I can now benefit from the work of these pioneers.

Why doesn't my doctor talk to me about preventing heart attack?

If the means to "turn-off" heart disease are already within our grasp, why don't most doctors tell you about it? Surely, if there were some medicine or health practice that could stop heart disease in its tracks, he/she would tell you about it!

Your doctor doesn't talk to you about heart attack because the concepts of silent coronary plaque detection, despite their power, have not yet reached mainstream consciousness among practicing physicians. Doctors can be very slow in abandoning deeply entrenched habits of practice and embracing new ways of thinking. Without heart scanning, your doctor is unable to predict who is going to have a heart attack and when among the vast majority of their patients.

Think about that for a moment. *Coronary disease is the number one cause of death in America, and most physicians do not know how to screen a seemingly well person for hidden heart disease.* You may, in fact, know of friends or acquaintances who passed their annual physical exam from their family physician, only to die or have a heart attack shortly afterwards.

Neal's story will illustrate this point:

I met Neal, an electrician, in the emergency room. He was in the midst of a large heart attack that was going to obliterate 50% of his heart muscle. His family physician had performed a stress thallium (a type of stress test) only one month before, when Neal felt perfectly fine. The stress test was negative: no chest pain, no EKG abnormalities, and the thallium images of coronary blood flow were normal. Neal was advised by his physician that his heart was in great shape and there was no risk for heart attack in the foreseeable future.

Three weeks later, Neal was lying on a hospital gurney, barely able to talk because of crushing pain in his chest. He answered my questions in brief phrases. He was terrified and bewildered. How could this be happening?

We got Neal through this near-death crisis and salvaged most of his heart muscle with an emergency coronary angioplasty and several stents. After he recovered, Neal asked the obvious question: "Why did I have a heart attack? My doctor said my stress test was fine! He said my heart was in perfect shape! Was the stress test wrong?!"

The stress test was *not* wrong. I reviewed the stress test and it was, indeed, completely normal. The problem was that it was *the wrong test*. Contrary to popular opinion, including that held by many physicians, stress testing is not an effective means of screening people without symptoms for the presence of coronary heart disease. This is such an important issue that I will repeat it: *Stress testing is not an effective method of uncovering hidden heart disease.*

Then why are stress tests performed? Are they worthless?

In truth, stress tests can be useful diagnostic tools, *but only when used appropriately*. People who go to the hospital *with symptoms*, particularly chest pain, can benefit by having a stress test to reproduce the symptoms. The physician needs to distinguish an impending heart attack from the pain of stomach ulcer, pleurisy (inflammation of the lining of the lungs from pneumonia), esophagitis (inflammation of the esophagus), gallstones, etc. If chest pain is provoked by walking on the treadmill during a stress test, this is suspicious for heart disease. The treadmill test (or a pharmacological equivalent) is often combined with a method of imaging blood flow to the heart muscle such as thallium, or methods to image heart muscle strength such as echocardiography (ultrasound). If there is poor blood flow to a specific segment of the heart's muscle, then a blockage in a coronary artery is present and your chest pain likely represents warning to a future heart attack.

Using a stress test to detect hidden coronary plaque in someone *without* symptoms is unlikely to uncover anything. This is because the majority of future heart attacks victims are walking around feeling just fine, yet have silent plaque in their coronary arteries. Heart attacks in these people are caused by rupture of a minor plaque, one that may be causing only 20 or 30% blockage, doesn't block blood flow, and is therefore *undetectable by any stress test.* Plaque rupture is a process that develops within minutes. Stress testing will not anticipate this event. (We will discuss this further in chapter 3.) What we really want to know is *how much plaque is present* in a well-appearing person.

The Track Your Plaque early detection concept

For up to 50% of heart attack victims, the first symptom of heart disease is their last. That means only around half the people with heart attacks actually survive long enough to make it to the emergency room. A heart attack is a potentially dangerous *terminal* event, not an early warning.

Track Your Plaque is built on the premise that heart disease should be detected early. We won't wait for symptoms to appear or catastrophe to occur. We will not wait for a stress test to show abnormalities, since only later phases of the disease are detectable this way. In Neal's case, had his coronary disease been identified before his heart attack, appropriate and powerful preventive action could have been taken. Maybe Neal's near-death episode could have been avoided.

We will measure hidden heart disease using methods to *detect coronary plaque,* before you have need of a stress test. This means looking for silent heart disease early, while you're feeling well, without symptoms, completely unaware of the plaque you conceal. As you will see, coronary plaque measurement is easy, inexpensive, precise, and provides far greater insight into your heart's future than any other risk factor or stress test.

A "yardstick" for heart disease

By far and away the easiest, most accurate, and inexpensive method to detect hidden heart disease is coronary artery calcium measurement. Given present day technology, your first choice in measurement of coronary calcium is through a heart scan using an electron-beam tomography (EBT) scanner or a multi-detector CT scanner (MDCT). These devices are becoming increasingly available. There are nearly 100 EBT scanners located throughout the U.S. Several new MDCT devices get underway every month, and they have already eclipsed the EBT in availability. What makes the EBT and MDCT heart scan approach so appealing is that it is *quantitative.* It is a precise measure of total plaque. The amount of plaque is reported to you as a "score", not just abnormal or normal. Just like the score in a basketball game, you can have low scores, intermediate scores, and high scores. You can think of the score as a yardstick for the quantity of plaque you have. That means we can not only identify plaque, but *track its increase or decrease.*

I feel great. Why should I worry about my heart?

Why can't you just wait for some tell-tale sign to appear, some symptom to tell you that heart trouble is ahead? Why look for heart disease while you're feeling great?

The reality is that the vast majority of people with coronary heart disease are *asymptomatic:* no symptoms of chest pain, arm pain, fatigue, breathlessness, etc.—yet dangerous heart disease can be present.

Let me tell you about Roger:

Roger is a 61-year-old construction worker, retired just several months earlier. It was his 11-year-old granddaughter's birthday, and he was about to treat her to a new bicycle at a department store. In her excitement, Roger's granddaughter raced through the store parking lot. When she turned to look at her grandfather, she saw him collapse face first on the parking lot pavement. The 11 year old yelled for assistance. A bystander turned Roger over, found no pulse, and initiated CPR. Roger's clear thinking granddaughter called to a store employee to dial 911. The EMT squad arrived within several more minutes. The ambulance ride to the nearest hospital was only seven minutes through light traffic, but Roger's heart stopped five times en route. The EMT personnel riding with him defibrillated his heart each time. They also inserted an endotracheal tube to ventilate his lungs. On arrival in the ER, an EKG showed an ongoing heart attack, in this case an inferior myocardial infarction, or a heart attack involving the underside of the left ventricular heart muscle. Roger was then stabilized briefly and again transported to an urban hospital 10 miles away where a full cardiac program was available. By this time, however, Roger became comatose.

Ten days later, after an urgent cardiac catheterization and stent to open the occluded artery and much hand-wringing by Roger's family, he recovered. But it was 10 days of not knowing whether Roger had sustained significant brain damage due to the multiple times his heart had stopped. His family spent countless hours at his bedside with Roger maintained on a ventilator, not responding to their presence.

Thankfully, Roger fully regained his mental function. Later during his recovery in the hospital, I asked him if he had any warning symptoms prior to his cardiac arrest and heart attack. Despite his ordeal, Roger had clear recollection of the events just up to collapsing on the parking lot pavement. He'd had absolutely no warning. In fact, he'd worked vigorously outdoors just the day before, clearing heavy brush on his land. He'd cut, sawed, swung an ax, raked debris and sweated, all without chest pain, breathing difficulties, or other abnormal sensations. Roger was extremely fortunate. Without the prompt action of everyone involved, especially his granddaughter and the bystanders outside the store, Roger's life would have ended without warning.

Roger suffered the consequences of a process that had built up over *decades.* Even in the last few moments, he was afforded no warning whatsoever, despite his own sort of "stress test" of heavy work.

Not everyone is as lucky as Roger. People who suffer a cardiac arrest in the field, i.e., in the community and not in the hospital, have less than a 1-in-10 chance of walking out of the hospital with their mental function preserved.

Given the fact that coronary heart disease will cause the death of one of every two males and one of every three females, it is a very real possibility in *your* life. If you followed conventional guidelines (of the sort likely used by your doctor), your heart disease will probably not be detected until symptoms develop or you suffer your first heart attack. You're feeling fine one moment, then seized by a choking sensation or chest pain, then drop, and it's all over. It can be just that quick. People die while exercising, while at work, watching television at home, or in their sleep.

Many people, including doctors, fool themselves into thinking that if heart disease develops, they will be provided some warning sign like chest pain or breathlessness. Then they can seek help and have the right things done. This is wishful thinking. The fact is that this very common disease strikes without warning and can kill you within minutes. Common sense should tell you that waiting to receive some warning of impending danger is just plain crazy.

"Maybe *I don't want to know* that I have hidden heart disease!"

People sometimes think that discovering hidden coronary plaque is like being given a death sentence. They'll say things like "Just do a bypass and let me forget about it!", or "I can't deal with this. You mean I could have a heart attack at any moment?!"

I regard these people as victims of hospital marketing and media. They have been brainwashed into thinking that any degree of coronary plaque means they need to submit to the technological know-how of the medical system. This is nonsense. It is foolhardy to *not* know whether you have hidden plaque, especially if you don't want to know simply out of fear. In reality, you and I can live perfectly happily with coronary plaque, provided it is not growing or active. We want to keep our plaque stable, not growing, not erupting. It is actively growing plaque that is heart attack prone. We want to arrest and perhaps shrink plaque to provide the reassurance we need to keep plaque from harming us.

When it comes to heart disease, ignorance is *not* bliss. Knowing whether you have hidden plaque can be the spark that ignites a powerful prevention program to keep you out of the hospital, keep you safe with your family, free of heart attack and symptoms. **Track Your Plaque** is a program of *self-empowerment* that returns control of your heart back to you.

Plaque grows over *decades* before heart attack

Not a week passes by that I don't hear about someone in my community dying suddenly from heart disease, and the victim and family had no inkling whatsoever that it was coming. I'm sure that you have friends, family, and acquaintances who've suffered similar fates. It's everywhere and it happens all the time.

The tragedy is that coronary heart disease requires *decades* to develop. If you were to have a heart attack and die at age 55, you didn't develop heart disease for the first time at age 53 or 54. It probably began in your *childhood,* and was readily detectable at age 40. Let me re-emphasize that point. Heart disease is *readily and easily detectable* 10, 15, or 20 or more years before it strikes you down. This is precisely the time when you and I should have our hidden plaque identified.

Some critics argue that providing warning to people years before danger is giving healthy people a disease, creating a class of what physicians call the "worried well". The **Track Your Plaque** experience has shown, however, that the more time you are afforded to take preventive action, the more powerful your results in preventing dangerous phases of heart disease in your future. This is, after all, a potentially fatal disease, not a sore back or bunion.

It is also key that the right people take action. Not everybody is at risk for heart attack and not everybody needs to engage in vigorous prevention. You should invest in a program of potent and effective prevention only if you are truly at risk. It's wasteful of your time and money and wasteful of our country's economic resources to prevent a disease you might never have. We should focus our efforts on those who will truly benefit.

How will *you* die?

It's a morbid exercise and may make you uncomfortable. Just for a moment, let's consider this question. Statistically speaking, how will you die?

The likelihood that you die of coronary heart disease is over 40%. That is, of all the reasons that humans die—cancer, infection, car accidents, inflammatory diseases like lupus, inherited and congenital diseases, degenerative diseases (diseases of "wear and tear")—coronary heart disease essentially equals all other causes *combined*. It's an easy bet. The overwhelming likelihood is that you and I will die of heart disease.

What if I then told you that we have a treatment that will reduce your risk of dying from heart disease, having bypass surgery, or having a heart attack by 35%? If you're a rational person, I would predict that you'd ask, "Why only 35%?!"

This is the premise of the National Cholesterol Education Program (NCEP) Adult Treatment Panel (ATP) guidelines. These are the guidelines designed by authorities on cholesterol for your physician to follow. NCEP has been responsible for the formidable task of interpreting the huge quantity of scientific and clinical data on cholesterol and distilling it down to an easily understandable format usable by the general practitioner. They've done a great job of accomplishing their goal. Cholesterol treatment is now an everyday practice in just about every family physician's office.

The NCEP guidelines are built on the concept that identifying people with high LDL ("bad") cholesterol, followed by treatment to lower LDL cholesterol, is an effective method of reducing heart disease risk. The NCEP panel is comprised of conscientious and dedicated physicians charged with the daunting job of drafting guidelines for broad consumption that won't bust the national budget, keep drug manufacturers happy, and yet provide useful advice for the practicing physician—generally well-intended concepts.

There are several serious flaws to this approach. First of all, the guidelines are built on the assumption that risk factors like cholesterol values, a history of diabetes, high blood pressure and smoking can tell us whether you will have heart disease or not. As you will see later in this book, trying to use risk factors to predict whether you have heart disease is a miserably deficient method. The majority of people with heart attacks have average cholesterol values, for instance. Secondly, a 35% reduction in the risk of heart disease is simply not good enough. If I told you that I had a cancer treatment that was 35% effective, would you be satisfied? Of course you wouldn't. While **Track Your Plaque** is not 100% effective—few things are—available data suggest that reductions of 80 to 90% in the likelihood of heart attack are very possible.

The NCEP approach also advocates very broad treatment of people with high cholesterols. The problem with this approach is that many people will need to be treated in order to prevent just one heart attack. For instance, in the widely publicized Scandinavian Simvastatin Survival Study (4S), a clinical trial that involved over 4000 patients over five years, one heart attack was prevented for every 20 people treated with the cholesterol-lowering agent, simvastatin (Zocor). That means that, in this five year time period, 19 people were treated but obtained little or no benefit.

Wouldn't it make more sense to precisely identify who is at high risk for heart attack and focus treatment just on those people? Perhaps we would be more effective by concentrating our energies on the people who are truly at risk. If you are destined to be among the unlucky 40% who die of heart disease, we'll establish this right from the start.

Rather than a 35% reduction in your risk for heart disease, our goal is far more ambitious: *eliminating* the risk of coronary heart disease in your lifetime.

But I eat healthy and exercise and I feel great!

Famous last words. That's precisely how I felt about myself, too. I followed a strict low-fat diet, avoided processed foods, and tried to jog or bike at least three to four times a week. Even when I pushed myself pretty hard, I had no chest pain or breathlessness. Yet, my coronary plaque *tripled* in the space of 18 months before I started applying **Track Your Plaque** principles to myself.

Tom provides another good example:

Tom is an architect. He's also become a good friend and I value his clever obser-vations. Tom is a perfect example of someone who did everything right yet still developed heart disease. Tom first came to me after he'd undergone a heart scan which revealed a high score of 385 (normal is zero), in the worst 1% of men his age. (We will discuss what these numbers mean in chapter 4).

At first, Tom was upset. He was 52 years old and in perfect physical shape. I mean perfect. If not running marathons, he biked 100 miles a day, easily passing men 20 years younger. He'd also been a vegetarian for 20 years and had never smoked. Tom adhered to this highly disciplined lifestyle because of his Dad's heart attack at age 53. His family physician had repeatedly complimented him on his favorable cholesterol values.

Ordinarily a calm man, Tom's face was red with frustration when we first met. "How could this possibly happen?! You can't be telling me to exercise harder! How can I eat any better? The test is wrong!"

I allowed Tom to calm down and told him that, unfortunately, the test was not wrong. Even extreme physical conditioning cannot guarantee protection from heart disease. It turned out that Tom had five reasons for heart disease, all relatively easily treatable reasons. Although Tom had been under the care of a very good physician, none of these abnormalities had been previously identified. He's been in the program for two years and doing well. He's just completed a cross-country biking trip and continues feeling great—and now he's safe.

It helped Tom to know that, had he not followed his healthy lifestyle, he would have had his first heart attack years earlier.

A great many of us, including myself in the past, walk around fooling ourselves into believing that we do such and such and therefore don't have to worry about heart disease. That's exactly what you're doing: fooling yourself. It is pure fantasy to believe that a diet low in fat, or a vegetarian diet, or even an extreme exercise program like Tom's can eliminate heart disease. These practices may *reduce* your risk (and the wrong diet may *increase* your risk), but for many of us, the genetic causes of heart disease will eventually reveal themselves. That's one of the areas where **Track Your Plaque** can help.

Aren't women different?

It is common for women's symptoms of active heart disease to be misperceived because of their tendency to have "atypical" symptoms, unlike men who are more likely to have straightforward chest pressure.

You will find that the distinctions between men and women melt away with the superior technology and simple three-step approach of **Track Your Plaque**. For one, the precise measurement of coronary plaque erases doubt over whether heart disease is present or not, regardless of whether you're a man or a woman. The amount of plaque you have is also viewed in light of your sex and age. Women are compared to women, men compared to men, and all stratified by age. A 43 year old woman, for instance, will be compared to other women her age, not 70 year old men. Likewise, in-depth understanding of the causes of heart disease provides *individual* insight free of sex bias. In short, the techniques used in **Track Your Plaque** can be the great equalizers in the male/female controversy, and you will find useful information in this program whether you're a man or a woman.

A program for life

Once you've begun your own **Track Your Plaque** program, can you go right back to old habits, hoping that the initial benefits will hold? Unfortunately, no. Old habits will revive quiescent plaque and reactivate the lipid/lipoprotein and genetic patterns that created plaque in the first place, and you'll be right back where you started. Roy's story will illustrate:

Roy was one of the early participants in the program. He came to me because of a high coronary calcium score and, as a result, Roy made substantial improvements in diet, began exercising, and added several supplements and prescribed medications. He did exceptionally well for the first 18 months of the program. Then Roy went through an unexpected and very traumatic divorce that left him emotionally devastated. He left his job without warning, packed a few belongings and got in his mobile home and drove west, drifting from town to town. After about a year of aimless wandering, Roy thankfully regained his perspective on life and turned around. Roy eventually returned to the office and related this sad story. In his despair, Roy had stopped all the treatments he'd begun and neglected the lifestyle changes. So we agreed to start with a reappraisal of his disease by repeating a heart scan. In the year since Roy stopped his treatments, his heart scan score had ballooned by 100%—he had doubled *the amount of plaque in his arteries.*

I've witnessed similar and frightening rates of disease growth in other people when the proper preventive strategies were not followed. **Track Your Plaque** is therefore not a one time "quick-fix", but a lifelong program for health.

How does Track Your Plaque fit into your life?

Track Your Plaque is primarily designed for people *before* heart attack and major heart procedures. Part of the reason for this is that the preventive and regressive efforts we will discuss can take months to years to take effect. A person who develops progressive or unstable symptoms of heart disease (rapidly progressing to a full heart attack) lacks sufficient time to take full advantage of these principles. As powerful as **Track Your Plaque** treatments are, they do not halt the progression to heart attack once this process is near completion. If you are having symptoms of chest or arm pain, or breathlessness, you may not be ready for this program. You may need the testing facilities provided by your doctor or hospital first, before you can safely consider these strategies.

Or, perhaps you're the kind of person who requires the reassurance of a hospital, people in scrubs and masks, and glitzy marketing. **Track Your Plaque** might not provide you with the kind of support you require. I may be critical

of hospital marketing, but I do not underestimate its power to influence people. Some people just need this sort of "legitimizing" presentation of their
healthcare, and independent, self-empowering practices may not suit you. If
you think that this may apply to you, I'd still encourage you to read on to
acquire a healthy dose of skepticism.

On the other hand, the earlier you start your program, the more power you
will have over your future. Preventing heart disease is a lot like saving for
retirement. If you start at age 35, saving a little at a time will yield a comfort-
able nest egg. Start at age 60, and you've got to scramble to reach the same goal,
or it might not be possible at all. The same holds true for inhibiting progression of coronary plaque.

What if I already have heart disease?

What if you've already had heart disease identified? Perhaps you've had a
coronary bypass surgery, or an angioplasty or stent, or you've had a heart
attack. Is it too late? Can you still benefit from this program?

Track Your Plaque is *best* suited for people who have not yet had these procedures, since the process of scoring your disease is distorted by bypass grafts
and stents. (We'll discuss why in chapter 4.) The rest of the program can still be
helpful to you. Shockingly, the great majority of people who have undergone
major heart procedures, despite having a proven dangerous disease, are often
provided little or no preventive counseling. These are the people who would
benefit the most from a vigorous effort in identifying the causes of their disease,
followed by specific treatments for each cause.

If you've already had a heart attack but have *not* received a stent or bypass
operation, then you are *ideally* suited for Track Your Plaque. You are farther
along the path of coronary disease than the usual asymptomatic participant in
Track Your Plaque. But the benefits can be just as great or greater. The scoring
process that is difficult following bypass surgery or stents can still be performed and play a part in your program. Likewise, lipoprotein testing to pinpoint the cause of your disease can provide you with lifesaving information.

How do I know Track Your Plaque is for me?

If you're a smoker, this book is not for you, at least not until you quit. No
program will fully overpower the negative effects of smoking. I've seen people
who did everything else right yet continue to smoke, and the quantity of coronary plaque doubles in a year's time. Smoking, even just a few cigarettes a day,

so overwhelms all your positive efforts that growth of your coronary plaque is inevitable. You've simply got to stop smoking to gain control of your plaque.

If you're looking for a quick answer—a special diet, a nutritional supplement, a prescription medicine—that "cures" you of heart disease and then you're done, you will not find your answer in this book. People with this attitude often don't take their risk for heart disease seriously. They don't participate in the learning process, are unwilling to make lifestyle sacrifices that may be necessary, and want to be told what to do but not participate in the decision making process.

On the other hand, people who succeed in **Track Your Plaque** tend to be motivated by learning and searching for self-empowering methods to preserve health. They recognize that health does not come in a single pill or diet, but grows from a combination of healthy habits. They understand that heart disease is a complex process with causes that vary from individual to individual, and that treatment and prevention also need to be individualized. This program appeals to people who are not content following the footsteps of their parents or other family members with heart disease, won't accept the inevitability of heart disease, and are willing to invest time and energy to create their own heart disease-free future.

Tracking your plaque is effective and not all that difficult. It cannot be distilled down to a single diet or pill. It is a comprehensive program that will require some effort, including a search for local resources in your area to assemble your own program. But the rewards can be great: prevention of a dangerous heart attack and avoidance of major heart procedures, potentially for a lifetime. Once you see the details and perhaps experience the results, I believe that you will agree that this is a far more rational way to approach the terribly common specter of heart disease in your life.

Summary

We have experienced a confluence of technological development that now makes early heart disease detection and prevention a practical reality. Despite the alarming epidemic of heart disease and its catastrophic consequences, the concept of early heart disease detection has not yet reached mainstream medical practice. **Track Your Plaque** can show you how you can begin to take advantage of new technologies and incorporate them into a powerful program of heart disease prevention.

Chapter 2

Your life is worth $60,853*

* Average cost of a coronary bypass surgery (American Heart Association, 2001)

Hospitals are in the business of heart disease.
You are in the business of prevention.

Ray was no newcomer to the hospital.

Ray survived his first heart attack 15 years ago that ruined a Caribbean vacation and forced him into early retirement at age 57. Since then, Ray has endured two heart bypass procedures, carotid surgery, five heart catheterizations, nine hospitalizations, and has graduated from cardiac rehabilitation classes after each of his bypass surgeries. Every time Ray goes to the hospital, he fears he'll end up with another heart catheterization if not another bypass.

Most recently, Ray was admitted to evaluate breathlessness he'd experienced while climbing stairs. A heart catheterization was being planned, no doubt. A review of Ray's medical history revealed that he has consistently received prompt, expert attention—Ray has never complained about the quality of his hospital care. What is surprising about his record is what is missing. Here was a 72 year old man who'd survived major and life-threatening events and procedures, yet not one comment had been made in his charts by his physicians about why Ray had such aggressive vascular disease. Not one. Ray's heart disease ended his productive work life, drastically impacted his personal life, and resigned him to a future of hospitals and procedures. The need for more procedures went unquestioned, yet virtually no thought was given to finding out the "why" of his disease.

Ray's story is, unfortunately, quite commonplace. Once you enter the hospital cardiovascular system, there is often no turning back, and your life can become a yo-yo of back and forth for more and more procedures. Over 25% of all bypass surgeries performed in the U.S. are so-called "re-do" procedures, bypass surgery for people who have undergone a prior operation several years earlier. The path for your future is inexorably established with more procedures, more hospitalizations.

"Coronary disease is a deficiency of polyethylene"

Back in 1990, I attended a large conference for cardiologists. This was the heyday of coronary balloon angioplasty, when we were all tantalized by the ability to open blockages in coronary arteries by inflating small balloons, or coronary angioplasty. One of the main speakers was a flamboyant cardiologist from Australia, a sort of "Crocodile Dundee" of cardiology. He joked that, because many coronary blockages were so readily opened with balloon dilatation, coronary disease could be regarded as a "deficiency" of 16 mg of polyethylene. (The balloons used were made of polyethylene.) I laughed along with my colleagues. Today, I believe this attitude remains the essence of the practicing philosophy of many physicians. Heart disease is a *procedural* disease best managed with hospital procedures like angioplasty and bypass surgery—period.

I have hundreds of patients who came to me because the only solution offered by their cardiologist was to perform a heart catheterization to determine the "need" for angioplasty, stents, and bypass surgery. If you turn out not to need a procedure, you are consigned to "medical therapy", which for a cardiologist means medicines like nitroglycerin, beta-blockers, and calcium channel blockers, which simply eliminate spasm in diseased arteries (arteries with plaque are very prone to spasm) and allow the arteries to dilate, or relax. Beta-blockers work by decreasing the heart's sensitivity to the body's adrenaline (epinephrine) and reduces blood pressure, making anginal chest pains less bothersome. Yet these medical therapies have little or no effect on the growth of plaque. With the exception of beta-blockers, these treatments also do not reduce risk of future heart attack. Medical therapy is, in fact, a miserable failure in reducing the relentless progression of coronary plaque growth.

Patients intuitively understand the concept of *regression* of coronary plaque. The idea that plaque can somehow be reduced or eliminated is very appealing. Talk to your neighborhood cardiologist, however, and you will find that plaque regression is not even part of his/her vocabulary. The idea is completely foreign because of their focus on ballooning, stenting, atherectomizing (cutting out) plaque through invasive procedures, or sending you to the operating room for a bypass procedure.

The hospital with the most bypass surgeries wins!

We live in an age when hospitals measure success by the number of coronary bypass surgeries they perform. Incredibly, it is still easier to get a bypass operation than it is to get good information on heart disease prevention. In the city where I live, there are billboards on the highways advertising bypass surgery. Selling bypass surgery nowadays is no different from selling cars, furniture, or televisions. It is a profit-driven enterprise whose success is measured by the volume of procedures sold.

Have you seen the TV commercials produced by hospitals? A man stumbles into the emergency room, clutching his chest. He's having a heart attack. Hospital staff in scrubs and masks pounce on their helpless patient. The camera pans to the tense eyes of the patient as he bids a tearful goodbye to his wife. The next scene shifts to the patient now beaming, congratulated by family and staff, and being wheeled out of the hospital after his successful coronary bypass operation.

Scenes like this are broadcast everyday by hospitals, eager to showcase their high-technology and track record of major cardiac procedures. Hundreds of millions of dollars, in fact, are spent annually to get these messages to you. Hospitals run ads to make sure you know about their successful, high-tech programs, but it's also to ensure a continuing stream of revenue from this huge growth industry called cardiac care.

When I travel, I am amazed by the uniformity with which this message is promoted. In city after city, from New York to San Francisco, you see ads everywhere, boasting of the strengths of one program or another. Physicians are often featured in "interviews," urging patients to come to their hospital for heart procedures. This constant media blitz is hugely expensive.

Cardiac care is big business. As a nation, we spend over $226 billion on cardiovascular care per year (American Heart Association, 2004). Annual hospital revenues for bypass surgery total in the neighborhood of $31 billion. Thirty percent of most hospitals' revenue and 50% of profits are from cardiac care. Heart disease and high-tech heart care to a hospital is like the Accord is to Honda, or Windows is to Microsoft—it's a hot seller.

There is substantial incentive for doctors to push patients through the cardiovascular procedure machine. There is, of course, the direct incentive provided by generous insurance reimbursement to physicians for performing these procedures. Every patient can mean thousands of dollars in income. It is interesting that, in states like California where the physician reimbursement for heart catheterization, angioplasty, and bypass surgery has been substantially slashed, the volume of procedures performed has dropped also. The disease itself hasn't changed. Read between the lines—the conclusion is obvious.

Less obvious are the indirect incentives provided to physicians who perform the most hospital procedures—access to equipment and staff, being featured in hospital marketing to achieve local notoriety, invitations to participate in decision-making committees, etc. High volume practitioners are often paid tens or hundreds of thousands of dollars for their referrals, often disguised as a "salary" or "retainer" to perform some administrative or consultative service. The results are a collusion to maintain high profit hospital business and grow market share. Arrangements like these are more common than you think.

If you were a hospital administrator, you would be under considerable pressure to sustain and build this engine of growth. Your job would be to capture more of this market. You would spend more and more money on flashy TV ads, billboards, and radio; try to win the allegiance of busy doctors; even disparage your competitors.

I have sat in many meetings attended by hospital administrators, cardiology and cardiothoracic surgery colleagues, and outside consultants, all to plan strategies for growth in cardiac care revenues. The question is always the same: "How do we increase the number of heart catheterizations, coronary angioplasties, and coronary bypass surgeries in our hospital?"

Prevent heart disease? You must be kidding!

Goodbye, St. Elsewhere!

Let's face it: the days of charitable hospitals devoted to the public good without interest in profit are long over. The healthcare industry, cardiovascular care in particular, is a *profit-driven enterprise* that uses all the tools of the business world: marketing, media relations, cultivating customers (physicians), growing their volume of product (patients), and increasing market share.

Hospital staff are the unwitting participants in this deception. When I discuss **Track Your Plaque** concepts with hospital nurses, technologists, and administrators, they are completely unaware of alternatives to acute hospital care. Many find these ideas personally appealing, but the pressures and incentives of the hospital are too hard to resist. After all, they've spent years training to do their jobs, and their salaries are paid by the hospitals providing these services.

Prevent heart disease? That's just not what hospitals do.

Well, it doesn't have to be this way. Given the proper tools, you can take control your future. As slick as hospital marketing can appear, as smooth as the process of bypass surgery is made to look, there are alternatives—*powerful* alternatives. If you are destined to have a heart attack in your future, the means to identify this potential can be made today, easily and painlessly. The therapeutic tools that prevent heart attack are also available right now. You just have to know where to look. **Track Your Plaque** can tell you where.

Fighting City Hall?

Following the **Track Your Plaque** principles is not all that difficult. You may, however, have a tough job ahead countering the skepticism of those around you. If you follow the principles in **Track Your Plaque**, you will begin thinking about how heart disease can be identified and measured, arrested and perhaps regressed ("reversed") in a world driven by hospital procedures.

You may encounter skepticism or even opposition from your doctor when you discuss some of the **Track Your Plaque** concepts. Should you talk to a cardiologist, he/she will more than likely scoff at the idea that coronary plaque can be controlled and regressed.

When I first set out to persuade my colleagues that there was a better way to approach coronary disease, I got the cold shoulder. After all, I was proposing to essentially "turn-off" coronary disease. Coronary procedures like heart catheterizations and angioplasties fill most of the day for a cardiologist. I encountered disbelief that coronary disease could ever be controlled with something less mechanical than a polyethylene balloon or metal stent. Many also pointed out that there was simply no money in prevention.

I pled my case to several hospitals in the area and asked them to consider supporting a program to help more broadly disseminate the ideas practiced in **Track Your Plaque**. Once again, I encountered glazed eyes and puzzled looks on the part of the hospital administrators and medical leadership. The concept of prevention, I painfully learned, is not one likely to be wholeheartedly adopted by hospitals. They are, after all, in the business of sickness, not wellness. Most hospitals do have programs in cardiac rehabilitation, which provide counseling and supervised exercise for patients after bypass surgery or heart attacks. That's about as far as it goes. I continue to hope that hospitals will eventually embrace the idea of a more comprehensive approach that addresses heart disease in the decades before procedures are required, but you are highly unlikely to get this kind of information from them today. If it doesn't contribute to their bottom line, then it just doesn't make sense for them.

Don't misunderstand my point. There are many times when high-tech, invasive care provided in hospitals is necessary. Centers that handle high volumes of these sorts of patients generally do it well and provide excellent service. Many lives have been saved and understanding of heart disease advanced. These services are often provided by capable, well-trained nurses and physicians who truly care about patients and are conscientious about the quality of their work. If you're taken to the hospital with unstable chest pain or an ongoing heart attack, it would be crazy to talk to you about detection of early disease and regression of plaque at that point. You need the services of a well-equipped, well-staffed hospital—no doubt about it.

Times are changing. Heart disease prevention has gotten a lot easier. It's no longer necessary to feel like you're fighting a losing battle against City Hall. All the new and exciting technologies we will discuss—heart scanning, lipoproteins, nutritional supplements, etc.—have become widely available. **Track Your Plaque** is your guidebook.

A heart attack is the *failure* of prevention

Imagine the homes in your neighborhood were being destroyed by fires day after day. Wouldn't you demand to know why preventive efforts were not being followed? Isn't it better to *prevent* fires than to struggle to extinguish a blaze once it's enveloping your house? The same holds true for your heart.

We should stand up in revolt and loudly reject the notion that heart disease inevitably results in dangerous events treated with hospital procedures. We should regard every heart attack, every angioplasty, every bypass surgery not as a success, but as a *failure*—a failure to identify these people before catastrophe strikes, when preventive efforts may have completely halted disease years earlier. If heart disease requires decades to develop and if methods to detect it are already available, can't we apply the tools to help those of us who are interested, and terminate the process *years* before trouble starts?

Heart disease regression is not new

As we shift our focus from crisis management to early identification and control, we naturally begin to wonder whether it is possible to shrink plaque. Patients often ask, "Don't you have any Drano for my arteries?"

The concept of regressing, or shrinking, coronary plaque is not new. Early efforts at plaque regression date back to the 1970s when techniques for both measurement of plaque and treatment were primitive. Back then, clinical trials, such as those conducted by Dr. Blankenhorn at the University of Southern California, required coronary angiograms (obtained via heart catheterization) to assess the extent of plaque. The treatments used included medicines no longer in use. Remarkably, some patients in these ancient trials did indeed obtain modest regression of plaque. These efforts lacked two crucial ingredients:

precise methods to measure plaque and effective treatment tools to control it. (We will discuss why heart catheterization is a flawed measure of plaque in chapter 4.) The results that are now possible are far superior to early efforts because we now have the ability to precisely measure and track plaque, and the tools to reduce plaque are more effective—and they're getting better every day.

Didn't Dr. Dean Ornish already write a book about this?

Since the publication of his bestseller in 1990, "*Dr. Dean Ornish's Program for Reversing Heart Disease*", Dr. Ornish has appeared on television, spoken articulately about his experiences to both lay and professional audiences, and has tirelessly discussed how dietary fat can cause heart disease and how a low-fat diet can help control it. Dr. Ornish deserves great credit for popularizing the notion that diet, exercise, and relaxation strategies (specifically meditation and support group interactions) can have an impact on progression of coronary heart disease.

Dr. Ornish originally advocated a vegetarian diet with 8–10% of calories from fat (compared to 40–55% in the average American diet), and permits no caffeine or alcohol. More recently, Dr. Ornish has allowed the inclusion of fish. It is a strict program. Critics have argued that few people can adhere to such a program for any length of time, let alone a lifetime. Dr. Ornish did manage to show that, with intensive counseling and supervision, people could indeed stick to it. In his published data, presented as "The Lifestyle Heart Trial" in 1990, he reported in The New England Journal of Medicine how 28 participants managed to reduce the amount of plaque in their coronary arteries. He proved this by having participants, all of whom had advanced coronary disease (at least moderate blockages in two or three coronary arteries) undergo a heart catheterization at the start of the program and then again after five years in the program. The participants reduced the severity of their heart artery blockages from 40.0% to 37.8% (measured by averaging the percent blockage, or stenosis, at many sites along the arteries), compared to a control group (people with comparable amounts of coronary disease at the start but not enrolled in Ornish's program), whose blockages worsened from 42.7% to 46.1% over the same five year period.

What is remarkable about Dr. Ornish's experience is that this was achieved with lifestyle changes alone. People eliminated red meat, pizza, greasy fried foods, and sweets, and were counseled on how to eat creatively using only vegetables, fruits and whole grains. No medication was prescribed, nor were supplements used.

Given Dr. Ornish's public success and notoriety, isn't that the end of the story?

Not even close. Dr. Ornish is a pioneer in the use of lifestyle modification to reduce heart disease risk, but his program falls far short of eliminating the dangers of heart disease. Of the 28 participants in the Lifestyle Heart Trial, two participants required bypass surgery, two had heart attacks, eight had angioplasty, two died of heart attack, and 23 were hospitalized over the course of the five year trial. Though this represented about half the number of events that occurred in the control group, that's still an awful lot of trouble. We need to improve on this track record.

In the early years of my practice, I recommended an Ornish-type diet program to many of my patients. Hundreds of them enthusiastically followed the guidelines and liked the idea of being in personal control of their heart disease future. As I applied more sophisticated measures, however, I observed that only about 20–30% of my patients demonstrated a truly favorable response. An ultra-strict low-fat diet did indeed lower LDL ("bad") cholesterols in most (but not all) people, but there were adverse distortions of numerous other measures (HDL cholesterol, triglycerides, LDL particle size, HDL particle size, VLDL). In fact, when heart scan scores are used to track the course of plaque growth, the majority of people's heart disease worsened, though perhaps at a somewhat slower pace. Heart attack, the need for heart catheterization, coronary angioplasty, and bypass surgery still occurred.

I applaud Dr. Ornish for his efforts, but I believe we've come a long way from his preliminary experiences. In **Track Your Plaque**, we will apply new technology and new insights. We broaden our choice of therapeutic tools and heighten our chances of success. Not only do I believe that results will be significantly better, but part of this approach is to *prove* it with precise tracking of the disease.

The tools to identify heart disease and alter its course to prevent cardiac catastrophes are available today. Perhaps you'll deprive the hospital from profiting from your $60,853 contribution, but your life is worth lots more, after all. Let's go on. In chapter 3, we discuss how coronary plaque develops and how we can use this knowledge to easily and readily measure it.

Summary

The business of medicine drives the need for hospitals to generate more and more revenue generating procedures like bypass surgery. But booming growth in hospital procedures is evidence of the *failure* of heart disease prevention.

Our goal should be to avoid requiring the services of a hospital. We should shift gears from crisis management to early detection, prevention, and even regression of silent heart disease. This is the basic premise of **Track Your Plaque.**

Chapter 3

What your doctor didn't tell you about heart disease

Why measuring coronary plaque is the most important health test you can get.

Paul was the picture of health. At age 50, he was a lean, muscular biking enthusiast. He and his wife, Sue, an ICU nurse, seized every opportunity to take long biking vacations in the southwest, Europe, anywhere they could. Paul was just as driven in his work. He'd risen to president of a manufacturing company, working his way up over the 10 years since he'd started. His two children, 13 and 15 years old, were both doing well in school and, to Paul's delight, shared his love of biking outdoors, too.

Because of his key position in the company, Paul submitted to mandatory physicals every year. Paul did so willingly, as his father had died of a sudden heart attack at age 49, collapsing on the floor in the kitchen in front of the family when Paul was 16 years old. This carved an indelible impression on his memory. So Paul asked the examining doctor specifically about heart disease. When the doctor learned that Paul had just biked 60 miles the weekend before, he laughed. "You've got to be kidding! How much better can your heart get?" He did, nonetheless, have Paul undergo an EKG and a stress test, both of which were perfect. The exercise effort on the stress test, in fact, barely caused Paul to break a sweat, despite the fact that he nearly set records in exercise capacity. The doctor also said his cholesterol values were all good and no treatment was recommended. Paul was satisfied with the results, as was Sue. After all, as a seasoned ICU nurse, she'd seen countless heart attacks and post-op coronary bypass patients and felt she knew what to look for.

One month later, Paul left work a few minutes early to squeeze in a little biking in the neighborhood around home. He failed to return at the expected time. After

Paul was an hour late, Sue started worrying and got in the car to look for her husband, in case he'd gotten injured. She knew his route, a less-traveled country road they used to avoid traffic, as she'd ridden it herself many times. After only 10 minutes of searching, she spotted someone lying in an unnatural position off to the side of the road, a bicycle several feet away. She felt the panic rise in her throat. She leapt out of the car—yes, it was Paul. Within minutes of her call to 911, the paramedics arrived, but Paul's body was already cold.

The circumstances of Paul's unwitnessed death prompted an autopsy. The coroner's report: death from a sudden, massive heart attack with extensive and advanced coronary plaque in all three arteries of the heart.

Let's look at heart disease from a new perspective. Even better, let's start from scratch. For a moment, let's put aside the dramatic images perpetuated by much of the media and hospitals—personnel in scrubs and masks, patients in operating rooms, high-tech procedures, etc.

Let's instead think of heart disease as a process that is hidden in about *half* of all adults over age 35. That's half of your friends and neighbors, half of the people at work, perhaps your husband or wife, maybe even your teenage children. When present in its early phases, it won't endanger you, but it's there, growing silently and rapidly.

Too little, too late

The medical community has been successful in developing tools to manage advanced complications of heart disease: bypass grafting, pacemakers, internal defibrillators, implantable hearts, etc. These are sophisticated tools to treat cardiac catastrophes. But the disease is present for *decades* before the catastrophe.

Paul's death represents an obvious example of the failings of the system. The conventional answer for someone like Paul would be to make emergency defibrillators more available in the community, so that bystanders can resuscitate victims of cardiac arrest. Or, it might be to shorten the amount of time required for first responders (emergency medical technicians) to reach the scene and begin resuscitative efforts. These are important issues, but shouldn't we also identify heart disease *before* these cardiac catastrophes develop? And not just a week or two before, but *years or decades* before heart attack, congestive heart failure, heart rhythm disorders, death? If we could predict that you were likely to have a heart attack or die five years from now, then instructed you in how to effectively prevent this, wouldn't this be a smarter, more rational approach?

The first step of **Track Your Plaque** is determining whether or not you have coronary artery disease in the first place, even in its early stages. We should *measure* how much disease, or plaque, is present. In other words, we must be able to *quantify* the disease, not just provide you with a "yes" or "no".

A one-minute lesson in coronary anatomy

We all have three arteries that provide heart muscle with its own blood flow. These three arteries sit on the surface of the heart (thus their name, "coronary", meaning crown) with numerous branches that dive into the heart muscle itself. The three arteries are named the right coronary artery, the left anterior descending artery, and the circumflex artery. Think of these arteries as upside-down trees, in that they start with a trunk and branch into successively smaller branches until you reach the twigs.

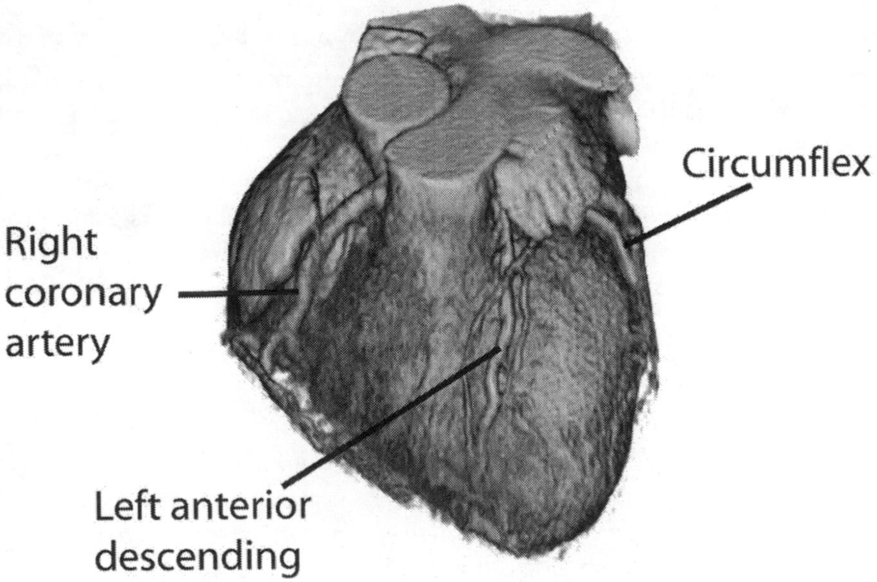

Circumflex

Right
coronary
artery

Left anterior
descending

Front-view of the heart showing the right coronary artery on the right (your left) and the left anterior descending in the front. The circumflex artery is seen on the far left (your far right). This image is a 3-D reconstruction of a real human heart using a technique called "electron-beam angiography" generated on an EBT scanner.

Cutting off the flow of blood at the level of the "trunk" of the artery, that is, in its uppermost portion, is most likely to result in a large quantity of heart muscle damage. Obstructing flow farther and farther downstream along the artery in its "branches" and "twigs" still causes damage but the amount of damage diminishes the farther out you go. A heart attack is exactly that: Obstruction of one coronary artery somewhere along its length. The higher up the artery the obstruction occurs, the larger and potentially more devastating the heart attack.

What are we measuring?

Exactly what "plugs up" coronary arteries?

As children, our arteries are flexible, thin-walled tubes, free of plaque. The walls of the arteries measure only a millimeter in thickness. As we age, various injurious factors (high blood pressure, nicotine, cholesterol-containing particles, oxidation, etc.) cause fatty tissue to accumulate in the arterial wall. Fibrous structural material, calcium (just like that in bone), and inflammatory cells also accumulate. The gruel-like material that results is called "atherosclerotic plaque." (*Athero* is derived from the Greek word for "gruel";-*sclerosis* means "hardening.")

Let's take an even closer look. We'll pretend that we have a handful of plaque taken from someone's arteries. We grind it up in a blender and then examine the contents. It certainly wouldn't be the prettiest mix, but we would have a fairly predictable combination of ingredients. There would be strands of fiber-like material (collagen) that provide strength to the plaque. Various cells would be found in our blender of plaque: muscle cells, fiber-producing cells, as well as inflammatory white blood cells. Cholesterol would be plentiful, since it is both a structural component of plaque, as well as an undesirable by-product that accumulates excessively. Calcium is also present, which is pebble-like and similar to the calcium found in bone. Curiously, calcium consistently occupies 20% of the overall volume of plaque—an observation that will prove very useful, as you will see.

It's one thing to blend up plaque that has been removed from someone's body. Can this mixture lining arteries be measured in a living, breathing person without submitting to procedures or tests that invade the body? That's the tricky part that has plagued physicians for years. For this reason, doctors resort to making *statistical predictions* on whether coronary plaque *might* be present based on cholesterol and other risk factors like blood pressure. What they are *not* telling you is whether or not you truly have plaque.

How can we measure coronary plaque?

Efforts to measure coronary plaque over the years have stumbled because of the heart's location within the chest, surrounded by the air-filled lungs. (Air obscures some imaging methods like ultrasound.) The heart is also in rapid motion. During each heart beat, some heart structures, including the coronary arteries, travel at a speed of two inches per second. (Part of the motion is rotational, or turning on an axis.) This is simply too fast for most imaging devices. On top of these hurdles, the coronary arteries are small, each measuring only about two to four millimeters in diameter. Imagine trying to snap a clear photo of a tiny bird flitting from tree to tree in a dense forest while you stand on the ground 100 feet away.

Technologies to image plaque within the coronary arteries are advancing at breakneck speed. Magnetic resonance imaging (MRI), for instance, is a clever method of visualizing internal organs by passing your body through a magnetic field. However, imaging plaque lining the rapidly moving coronary arteries is still impractical with this technology, mostly because MRI is still too slow for the moving coronaries. A few more years and this will likely become a viable choice.

One way to circumvent the limitations in coronary imaging is this: if we understand what plaque is made of, and if plaque components occur in fairly *consistent proportions*, we can then use *one* of the components of plaque to measure the total volume of plaque. Recall from our make-believe plaque-in-a-blender that calcium comprises 20% of the ingredients in plaque. The measurement of *calcium* can be used as an indirect, but highly reliable, measure of the quantity of plaque, since it occurs in a predictable proportion in plaque. This phenomenon can be used to image plaque with new computed tomography (CT) technologies. Recent developments in this area permit ultra-rapid, reliable, and inexpensive imaging of hidden coronary plaque. This approach has become very accessible, as well, with a suitable device within driving distance for nearly everyone in the U.S. For these reasons, the new CT imaging technologies are the method of choice for tracking your plaque. In chapter 4, we'll discuss everything you need to know about coronary calcium scoring on these new devices.

Heart disease is a disease of youth

How early in life does plaque develop? Does plaque first appear at age 40, or 50, or 60? No. *Coronary plaque first develops in our teens and twenties.* This became clear during the Korean War when young soldiers (average age 22 years old) who died in battle were studied at autopsy. To the surprise of the doctors performing the autopsies, three quarters of these young, seemingly healthy men had atherosclerotic plaque lining their coronary arteries, many of them advanced. These men had been engaged in extremely physically demanding battle and were obviously not suffering from chest pain or other symptoms.

This disturbing observation has been confirmed time and again, even with examination of *children's* arteries. The message is clear: coronary disease first develops when we are young and progresses over decades. This doesn't mean, of course, that children or teenagers need bypass surgery, nor does it mean that they will have a heart attack in their twenties. It does mean that the "seeds" of plaque are planted early in life and grow over the ensuing years.

Track Your Plaque—Hal

To illustrate this process, let's invent a hypothetical man we can follow from the beginnings of his coronary plaque as a teenager to his eventual heart attack.

Our make-believe man is named Hal, an average American. At age 18, Hal just graduated from high school and is healthy and in the best physical condition of his life. His coronary arteries at this point appear smooth and open. The only evidence of coronary disease is a mild thickening of the internal lining of all three arteries. Hal's life is filled with pizza and fast foods, hectic days, and nights with little sleep, but he feels great as he prepares to go to college.

Hal finishes college, lands a job, marries and has two children. Hal endures the pressures of work and family, but leads a relatively sedentary life. He rarely exercises except for playing with his kids or an occasional round of golf, and gains about 20 pounds. At age 30, Hal tips the scale at 202 pounds, the most he's ever weighed, although he wouldn't regard himself as obese. Outside of work stress, Hal feels pretty good. When we examine Hal's coronary arteries, he already has a thick lining of plaque throughout the entire arterial tree. In some areas, the plaque is as thick as two or three millimeters, even though the opening of the artery (or lumen) is also about three millimeters. In fact, if we compare the external diameter of Hal's artery at age 30 to that at age 18 (i.e., looking at the artery from its exterior), his arteries at age 30 are substantially larger. Hal's arteries have adapted to the accumulation of plaque by enlarging (a process called the Glagov phenomenon, or adaptive remodeling). This process permits plaque to grow without impinging on the path for blood flow. It means that, if Hal were to undergo a heart catheterization in his hospital, he would be told that he has no coronary disease. His arteries would be given a clean bill of health and appear completely "clean," because the internal diameter was still normal and the thick, extensive plaque in the artery wall was not detected. In reality, Hal's arteries are loaded with plaque, just disguised by the process of remodeling.

(Does the enlargement process protect Hal from heart attack? No, not at all. In fact, Hal's remodeled, enlarged arteries are *more* likely to cause heart attack. Blood flow is maintained, but the probability of sudden closure of his arteries has *increased*.)

Hal is now 40 years old. His kids are in their teens and Hal has advanced in his career. Although Hal has gained another 15 pounds—he now weighs 217—he still feels that he's in perfect health. After all, he feels fine, his energy is good, he doesn't smoke, drinks only occasionally, and he still manages to fit in a round of golf now and then and walk the neighborhood with his wife twice a week. Now Hal's coronary arteries are lined top to bottom with a thick layer of plaque. The process of enlargement has now been exhausted and any further accumulation of plaque begins to grow inward. At this point, if Hal had a heart catheterization, he would be told that he did indeed have some plaque, although the full extent of his plaque would be underestimated. He'd be told, "Your blockages are minor, so you don't need any stents or bypass surgery". The truth is that minor blockages are only the tip of the iceberg of extensive plaque lining the arteries. Still, Hal has no chest pain, no difficulty breathing, and is completely unaware of his coronary plaque.

Why are "minor" plaques dangerous?

Any coronary plaque has the potential to rupture. However, plaques more likely to rupture have several features:
1) "Pools" of semi-liquid fat, or lipid, with the consistency of toothpaste
2) Inflammatory cells
3) A thin-walled covering between the lipid "pool" and bloodstream

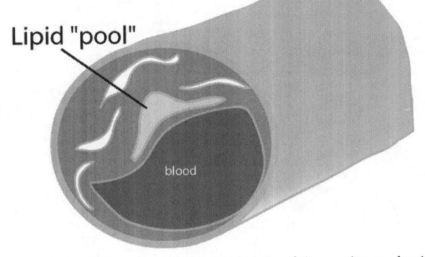

A plaque that is likely to rupture. Note the thin rim of tissue acting as a barrier between the lipid pool and blood (sometimes called a "cap"). The white unlabeled areas represent collections of calcium that can be used to measure total plaque volume. *The severity of blockage has little to do with the likelihood of a plaque rupturing.*

When ruptured, plaque contents are exposed to the blood flowing past and are powerful triggers of blood clot formation. The growing blood clot can completely occlude the artery and cut off blood flow, creating a heart attack, or myocardial infarction.

People accumulate not just one or two plaques but dozens, and they may cover nearly the entire length of the lining of each artery. Each and every plaque has some potential for rupture. So having many plaques poses substantial risk, since a single rupture can cause heart attack, even if it begins as only a 20% blockage.

Hal's doctor is concerned about Hal's mildly elevated LDL cholesterol of 144 and the fact that Hal's father suffered a fatal heart attack at age 59. He therefore suggested that Hal be screened for hidden heart disease by undergoing a stress test with radioactive imaging of his heart, a stress thallium. It's completely normal. Despite Hal's neglect of vigorous exercise, he exceeds the level expected for a man his age, he has no abnormal symptoms, his EKG doesn't show any abnormalities, and coronary blood flow is normal by the radioactive thallium images.

So Hal goes about his life, feeling just fine, yet harboring a growing burden of plaque lining his arteries. One day, Hal wakes up early with a vague ache in his chest. One of Hal's numerous coronary plaques has ruptured, or eroded its thin covering of tissue, exposing the plaque's internal contents of fat and cholesterol to the blood flowing past. The exposed material is a powerful instigator of blood clot formation. Within minutes, the clot grows and cuts off blood flow in the coronary artery.

Hal breathes deeply, moves around, hoping that this muscle or stomach ache will just go away. Over the next 10 minutes, it just keeps intensifying, becoming excruciating, the worst pain he's ever experienced. Hal's wife knows right away what's happening. Hal is having a heart attack. She calls 911. In the minute it takes to make the call, Hal has dropped to the floor. Hal's wife, panicking, tries to remember her class in CPR. The ambulance squad arrives 10 minutes later. They intubate Hal (insert an endotracheal tube in his throat for oxygen), perform CPR, and shock his chest. Even though they load Hal's body onto the gurney, still performing CPR, Hal's wife knows the truth: Hal is gone, just 50 years old.

Hal's tragic story is, of course, fictitious. But stories just like Hal's are an everyday reality. Little or no warning, no symptoms in the weeks or months leading to heart attack, dying suddenly—from a process in the coronary arteries that had been present since teenage years.

Hal's arteries as a child. No plaque is present. The artery is thin-walled and flexible.

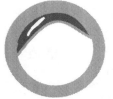

Hal's arteries at age 18. Plaque has begun to grow. Plaque (dark gray) contains cholesterol, supportive tissue, and inflammatory cells. Calcium (white) has started to appear, also.

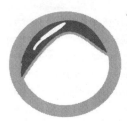

As Hal enters his 30's, plaque grows. The diameter of the artery increases to accommodate the growing plaque ("remodeling"). More calcium (white) accumulates, occupying 20% of plaque area.

Hal, age 36. Plaque has grown larger with more calcium, as well as scattered collections of fatty material (not shown). The arteries can no longer enlarge to accommodate growing plaque and the internal diameter gets narrower.

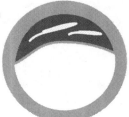

Hal, age 40. Plaque is extensive and lines the entire length of his arteries. There is active inflammation and lots of fat ready to "erupt". At this point, Hal's stress test is normal and a heart catheterization would show "mild blockages".

Hal just before his heart attack at age 50. Inflammation and fatty tissue make the plaque contents unstable. One day, these materials digest their way to the surface and become exposed to blood. A blood clot forms and blood flow is cut off. Hal suffers a heart attack. Had Hal undergone a stress test in the days or weeks before his heart attack, it may or may not have been abnormal.

Hal's coronary plaque from age 18 to 50 as it progresses from minor fat accumulation to extensive fat and calcium containing tissue. Remember that the three coronary arteries are each several inches long, and this process, represented in cross-section, develops along the entire length of the arteries.

Your stress test is normal—but you have heart disease!

Let's consider this for a moment. Hal had an advanced degree of coronary atherosclerosis, with plaque lining the entire length of his heart's arteries. Yet his stress test was normal. (Although Hal's story is, of course, fiction, this situation is exceedingly common.) How can that be? Don't doctors use stress testing to screen people for heart disease?

Unfortunately, the great majority of physicians in practice do indeed use stress testing in various forms to screen people without symptoms for heart disease. Even the American Heart Association (AHA) has issued policy statements that discourage this practice. The AHA recognizes that the majority of people with silent heart disease *will not be identified by stress testing*—the test will be absolutely normal. The AHA has also recognized that many people *without* heart disease will have *abnormal* stress tests, so-called "false-positives". (American College of Cardiology/American Heart Association 2002 Guideline Update for Exercise Testing.)

The most persuasive argument against stress testing is the observation made as long ago as the 1980s that, of every 100 people who have a stress test, about 10 will be abnormal. *The majority of future heart attacks and deaths will occur among the 90 people whose stress tests are normal.*

If you have undergone a stress test and were told that your heart was in great shape and there's nothing to worry about, you now know that this could be absolute nonsense.

Stress testing is, however, an effective method your doctor can use to understand symptoms. If you report an ache in your chest to your doctor, an EKG and a stress test can help understand whether the chest discomfort is an impending heart attack or hiatal hernia (when the upper stomach slides up and down through a hole in the diaphragm), esophagitis (inflammation of the esophagus), gallstones, etc., since a wide variety of disorders can cause similar symptoms.

Stress testing is based on the principle that, when plaque accumulates sufficient to obstruct blood flow through the artery (generally occluding the diameter of the artery by 70% or more), several things happen. A person may experience chest pain or breathlessness, the EKG may show specific abnormalities and, if the heart is imaged using radioactive materials or ultrasound (echocardiogram) during exercise, evidence for poor blood flow may be detected. Unless there is a *severe* blockage with reduced blood flow, a stress test will be normal. Recall from Hal's story that extensive plaque can accumulate in the artery walls without blocking blood flow because of the process of remodeling, or enlargement of the artery.

Who cares if you have silent plaque?

Many people ask, "If you have plaque in your coronary arteries that can't be detected by stress testing, so what? Are there any dangers from silent plaque"?

You bet there are. In fact, study after study through the late 1980s and 1990s demonstrated that, much to the surprise of many practicing cardiologists, the majority (>70%) of heart attacks originate from mild blockages of 20–50%. *These plaques don't block blood flow and don't cause symptoms.* They would not be ballooned, stented, or bypassed. Yet mild plaques pose the greatest risk and are undetectable by stress testing.

Should everyone considered at risk for heart attack then undergo heart catheterization to detect silent coronary plaque? (Don't laugh—this argument has actually had many proponents.) Catheterization greatly underestimates the amount of plaque in the wall of the arteries because of remodeling, just like Hal's arteries. Having performed several thousand heart catheterizations myself, I can tell you that, when x-ray dye is injected directly into the heart arteries, we fill the artery lumen (like the inside of a water pipe) and observe its contours. While this approach can show your cardiologist where the most severe narrowings are, it reveals nothing about the condition of the artery walls. In fact, the cardiologist cannot tell whether your arteries are severely thickened, lined with atherosclerotic plaque, or whether they are entirely normal. This test is also invasive, requiring catheters to be inserted into the leg or arm and navigated to the heart. Catheterization costs $8000–$12,000, even if done without admitting you to the hospital. Cost, potential danger, and imprecision make heart catheterizations an undesirable choice for screening purposes.

A technology called intracoronary ultrasound has helped make sense of the seeming disconnect between quantity of plaque in the artery wall and the severity of blockage. Intracoronary ultrasound is the closest thing to actually examining arteries as if they were right in the palm of your hand. In this procedure, an ultrasound probe is passed into a patient's coronary artery and highly detailed cross-sectional pictures obtained. Ultrasound studies have shown that the severity of blockage, say 50% or 90% by catheterization, has little to do with the amount of plaque present in the wall, and vice versa. (See diagram.) Often, portions of the artery that appear normal or minimally diseased by catheterization are actually loaded with plaque by ultrasound.

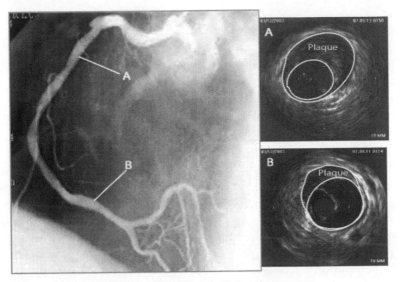

Cardiac catheterization does not reveal all the plaque
Cross-section A is from an area of mild blockage on the catheterization view, but is really filled with plaque when examined by intracoronary ultrasound. The area occupied by plaque, in fact, exceeds the path for blood to flow (smaller circle). Cross-section B is also from an area of mild blockage and intracoronary ultrasound does indeed show only a mild arc of plaque. The images made at catheterization do not necessarily reveal the true amount of plaque in the artery wall.

It is, therefore, the *amount of plaque* in the wall of the artery, *not* a reduction in the internal diameter, that determines risk for heart attack. (Cardiologists call this "plaque burden".) Whether a specific portion of an artery has a 10%, 30%, 50%, 70%, or even 90% blockage has very little to do with the heart-attack potential of this blockage. (An exception to this is when you are just on the verge of a heart attack and the artery is about to close. In this situation, a severe blockage may be properly judged to be the active source of trouble. This is more likely to be the case for people, for instance, in the emergency room with accelerating chest pain symptoms.) It is, however, the 90% blockage that is fixed (by ballooning or stenting) or is bypassed, as it can be a source of symptoms. All the other less severe blockages—of which there may be dozens—are not fixed yet pose substantial risk for heart attack because of their potential for rupture.

Just having plaque is bad enough!

I hope you now see that having *any* quantity of plaque in your coronary arteries is sufficient reason to be concerned that heart attack might be in your future. Keep in mind that, once plaque is established, it grows—and it grows rapidly. We used to believe that plaque growth was a slow phenomenon requiring years for significant worsening. Newer methods show frightening rates of growth. The volume of plaque in your arteries can easily *double* in a year.

Remember Paul, the business executive whose sad story opened this chapter? How could his life have been changed by following the simple concepts of **Track Your Plaque**? Let's see:

Paul passes his physical with flying colors. The doctor is still concerned about the history of Paul's father dying of a heart attack as a young man. Because of Paul's excellent fitness and absence of symptoms, rather than a stress test the doctor suggests that Paul undergo a scan to detect hidden coronary plaque.

Paul has his scan, requiring 10 minutes of his time. A call from the doctor follows. He tells Paul that he has extensive plaque in his heart's arteries, more than 90% of all men his age. At age 49, Paul has the coronaries of a 75 year old man. "Does this mean I have to have a bypass operation?" Paul asks with alarm. "No, absolutely not. It does *mean that a serious approach to prevention is needed and we need to begin right away. We will pinpoint the causes of your plaque and then correct them. Simple as that." A single series of blood tests reveals Paul's five causes of plaque and a treatment program is devised. Paul goes back to work and life with his family, sharing biking vacations together.*

Step 1 of **Track Your Plaque** is to measure coronary plaque. We therefore need a tool to do so reliably, easily, painlessly, at little or no risk, and inexpensively. We discuss this further in chapter 4.

Summary

The conventional approach to diagnosing coronary disease leaves the vast majority of people with silent heart disease undetected and unsuspecting, despite the fact that approximately half of all American adults over 35 harbor hidden coronary plaque.

Identification and quantification of coronary plaque potentially provides a powerful measure of future heart attack potential. Plaque accumulation is a process that begins early in life and develops over decades before heart attack. This means that silent coronary plaque can be detected years before catastrophe strikes when the proper tools are applied.

Track Your Plaque

Step 1

Chapter 4

Heart disease can be *measured*

A *"yardstick" for coronary plaque*

If you have hidden heart disease, is it still early in the process? How much time do you have before your cardiac catastrophe? Perhaps your heart attack is far in the future, say in 10 or 20 years, allowing you plenty of time to develop a powerful preventive program. Or, do you already have extensive plaque, and the burning fuse on this bomb is getting shorter until your heart attack next week or next month? Or, maybe you have absolutely *no* plaque, and you will *never* suffer a heart attack.

Obviously, these are crucial distinctions.

They are distinctions we *cannot* make by looking at your cholesterol or blood pressure, or by how your feel, your weight, even a stress test. You may feel fine. You don't experience chest pain, breathlessness, etc. You may have a "great" cholesterol, perhaps you've never smoked, and maybe you passed a stress test. You can still have plaque lurking silently in your heart's arteries, and it may be early or it may be extensive.

Let's take a hypothetical woman, Joan, with a LDL cholesterol of 143. She's 46 years old, a non-smoker, 15 lbs. overweight, with a family history of heart attack in her father at age 60. She feels perfectly fine and exercises moderately. Based on this information, can you tell me if Joan has heart disease or not?

I certainly can't, and neither can your doctor. Yet this is the dilemma doctors face every day, trying to decide who will have heart attack in future based on cholesterol values and other risk factors. For all we know, Joan may have extensive heart disease and is at potential risk for dying within the next year—or she may have no disease at all. Trying to extract this information out of cholesterol values is a useless exercise.

If we polled 100 people who suffered heart attacks, what do you think the average LDL cholesterol would be? You'd expect it to be high, wouldn't you? It's an important question. After all, these people experienced an event that carried nearly a 50% chance of dying. The average LDL cholesterol in this group would be 134 mg/dl. The majority of LDL cholesterols, in fact, would range from 80–180 mg/dl (National Health and Nutrition Survey III, 1988-1994). Compare this to the average LDL for the healthy U.S. population: 130 mg/dl. This means that there is substantial overlap in LDL cholesterols among people destined for a heart attack and those who will never have one. Does having an LDL cholesterol *greater* than 130 mean you are about to die of a heart attack? Does having an LDL *less* than 130 mean that you will never have a heart attack? The answer to both questions is no, of course.

Half of all heart attacks occur in people with LDL cholesterols below 134 mg/dl, half occur in people with LDL cholesterols above 134 mg/dl. The national guidelines for cholesterol treatment (National Cholesterol Education Program Adult Treatment Panel III guidelines, 2002) don't even suggest cholesterol lowering treatment for LDL at this level in the general population.

How can this be? If high cholesterol causes heart disease, how can you have coronary disease and heart attacks even with low cholesterols? How can we possibly identify people at risk for heart attack from this confusion?

Relying on cholesterol values to identify hidden heart disease is about as good as tossing a coin. If we decided to focus only on people with LDL cholesterols greater than 134, for example, then we'll miss half of all heart attacks. The same is true for other common measures, like the total cholesterol/HDL ratio. None of these values can distinguish, with good confidence, who will or will not have a heart attack.

Should we treat you to prevent a future heart attack—heads or tails?

Cholesterol does have its usefulness. Cholesterol levels are indeed *statistically* related in a graded fashion to risk of heart disease, i.e., the higher the cholesterol, the greater the likelihood of heart attack in your future. The Multiple Risk Factor Intervention Trial, or MR FIT ("Mister Fit"), demonstrated this principle. Among 12,000 participants, the MRFIT trial showed that the higher the total cholesterol, the higher the risk of heart attack, with the likelihood of heart attack in the people with the highest 25% of cholesterols three times that in the lowest 25%. About 40% of all heart attacks, however, still occurred in people with low total cholesterols below 240. There are also *many more people* with low or middle-range cholesterols than there are people with high cholesterols. As a result, there are just as many people with heart attacks who start with low cholesterol as there are with high cholesterols. So the higher the cholesterol, the higher the statistical risk of heart attack, but a significant number of heart attacks still occur at low or normal cholesterol values.

The widely publicized Framingham trial also illustrated this phenomenon. Thousands of residents of Framingham, Massachusetts were studied over a period of 20 years to discern what measures might predict heart attack. The Framingham researchers found that cholesterols of people who developed heart attacks overlapped with 80% of the people without heart disease. In other words, four out of five people fell into this large middle range of cholesterols, whether or not they developed heart disease. Extremely low total cholesterols of <150 had low risk (though not zero risk) for heart attack; extremely high cholesterols >300 had high risk for heart attack (three-fold higher). The overwhelming majority of people fell in between these extremes, and the greatest number of heart attacks were suffered by these people.

Using cholesterol testing to identify people with heart disease is like trying to predict who is going to die on a high speed freeway. If the likelihood of dying in an automobile accident on the highway tripled if you drove faster than 65 mph, does this help you decide who is going to die and who is not going to die in a highway accident? It does, but only in a vague statistical sense. These broad measures of risk help in analyzing large numbers of people. When you try to apply these rules to a specific individual, they utterly fall apart. Does driving 68 miles per hour mean you're going to die in a car accident? Does driving 62 miles per hour mean you will never die? Of course not. These observations are only *statistically* predictive.

So why not assume that *everybody* with LDL cholesterol above 100 has coronary disease and just initiate treatment? Or above 90? Or even 50?

The problem is that, the lower the LDL cut-point you use for treatment, the more people will be treated who will never have a heart attack. That could represent years of cholesterol lowering treatment at substantial cost, not to mention a small risk of side-effects as well, but without benefit. In addition, there are many other causes of heart disease besides LDL cholesterol. Instituting treatment for LDL cholesterol does not eliminate heart attack or other catastrophes.

The best risk factor of all is...

Is there a risk factor that, when present, predicts a high probability of future heart attack? A risk factor that can distinguish with great confidence who will or will not have a cardiac catastrophe in future? A risk factor that tells us whether you have extensive coronary plaque or no coronary plaque? Yes, the presence of coronary plaque. Let me say that again. The person at highest risk for heart attack (from a ruptured plaque) is the person who already has plaque. This is true regardless of whether LDL cholesterol is 92 or 192. This is because *coronary plaque is a measure of the disease itself.* If you think about this for a moment, it makes perfect sense. *The risk for rupture of a plaque occurs when there is plaque already present to rupture.* If you don't have any plaque, you can't rupture it. So it's not so much whether cholesterol is high or low, it's whether you have the necessary plaque to permit rupture.

A hint of this phenomenon was suggested as long ago as the 1970s and 80s in the Coronary Artery Surgery Study (CASS), when people who were told they had mild coronary disease (blockages of <50%) still suffered substantial risk of future heart attack and death, similar to people with severe degrees of blockage. Once again, *just having plaque* was a powerful predictor of future danger. Even today, people with mild blockages (<50%) are often wrongly told, "You only have mild blockage, there's nothing to fix. You don't need a bypass and your risk for heart attack is low." Unfortunately, physicians equate the lack of need for bypass (or stents) with mild and therefore inconsequential coronary disease. This is simply wrong. People with even mild plaque can have substantial risk for heart attack, not very different from people with severe blockages.

To illustrate the superiority of plaque measurement to cholesterol, let's compare the likelihood of heart attack in people with high cholesterols (say, total cholesterols above 300—really high) to people with high coronary calcium scores (and therefore with extensive plaque). High cholesterol (>300) raises risk of heart attack three-fold (compared to people with low cholesterol). The high calcium score raises risk as high as *twenty-fold* (when compared to zero scores). In other words, having coronary plaque identified is the most powerful predictor of future heart attack, a far superior predictor to cholesterol. In fact, very high scores (>1000) can predict a 25% per year risk of heart attack or death even when no symptoms are present and stress test is normal. *No cholesterol measure has this kind of power to predict the future.*

Having *no* detectable plaque, on the other hand, can tell us confidently who is *not* at risk for heart attack. Dr. Paolo Raggi, of Tulane University, has shown that the likelihood of heart attack in people with a heart scan score of zero is nearly zero. If you don't have coronary plaque, it is highly unlikely you have a heart attack. (There are rare exceptions—people who take cocaine or amphetamines, for instance, can experience heart attacks due to severe coronary artery spasm, even without prior plaque build-up.) In one of Dr. Raggi's recent studies of over 600 people, *one heart attack occurred in the group with a 0 coronary calcium score, while over 99% of the heart attacks occurred in people with measurable plaque (with abnormal heart scan scores).* Dr. Raggi also showed very clearly that the higher the score, the greater the likelihood of heart attack. No other risk factor can even come close to this kind of discriminatory value.

In short, the most powerful indicator of your future risk of heart attack (or needing bypass surgery, angioplasty, or stents) is having coronary plaque measured. This approach turns the whole world of cholesterol testing topsy-turvy. We will discard the idea of using cholesterol values as the first step to tell us whether or not you should be seriously considered for heart disease risk. If you've been told either that you don't have coronary disease based on low cholesterol, or if you've been told you likely have coronary disease based on high cholesterol, start all over again. Let's go straight to a measure of the disease itself: coronary plaque.

We therefore need an accurate means of quantifying *all* coronary plaque, both visible and hidden. We need to do so not just at one or two spots along the arteries, but *along the entire length of all three coronary arteries,* from top to bottom. The more extensive the plaque, the higher the risk for heart attack— *even in the absence of severe blockage.* The greater the quantity of plaque that lines your coronaries, the more opportunity there is for rupture that results in heart attack. Detecting and measuring coronary plaque is the crucial first step of the three steps of **Track Your Plaque.**

The plumber's dilemma

When you think about it, it might not be such an easy thing to do: precisely measure the amount of plaque lining three coronary arteries along their six-inch lengths, all while the heart is beating, concealed within the chest.

Imagine asking a plumber to assess the water pipes in your home and tell you just how much rust is lining them. Obviously, he can easily tell you that the pipe in the bathroom sink is leaking. Could he assess the internal condition of the entire length of the pipes in the house? Pretty tough.

What if another plumber came along and told you, "58% of the pipes in your home have an average of 1.6 mm of circumferential rust lining the internal surface, giving you a total of 7,890 cubic mm of rust. This is more severe than 90% of all other homes." In other words, this plumber precisely *quantified* the amount of rust present throughout the entire water pipe system. You now have a much better picture of the "health" of your plumbing. This is analogous to what we are trying to achieve in the coronary arteries. We would like to measure the health of the entire tree of arteries.

As discussed in chapter 3, many physicians still regard heart catheterization as the gold standard to diagnose coronary disease. Numerous studies have definitively shown that the blockages seen at catheterization greatly underestimate the true extent of plaque. More detailed (though still invasive) examination of the artery walls can be made with intracoronary ultrasound, which provides images in cross-section by passing a high-frequency sound emitting catheter along the length of each artery. Surprisingly, ultrasound reveals that the most extensive plaque frequently occurs in areas along the length of the artery *with no significant blockage*. Severe blockages are just the tip of the iceberg of a process that is far more extensive. The artery wall, in fact, can be *loaded* with abnormal plaque, yet the internal diameter appears normal. This would be like the first plumber who was only able to identify the sites of leaks—helpful information, but it tells you little about the overall condition of the pipes. You might even be misled to believe that, because you had no obvious leaks, your pipes were entirely free of rust.

Can plaque be measured in a living person?

Let's re-visit our hypothetical friend, Hal (chapter 3), before his fatal heart attack at age 50. You will recall that, at age 40, Hal already had a layer of thick plaque lining the length of all three of his coronary arteries from top to bottom. You'll also recall that Hal underwent a stress test (a stress thallium to assess the volume of blood flow) that was normal. Had he undergone a heart catheterization as well (needlessly, by the way), he would have been told "Hal, your arteries are in great shape. There are only a few minor blockages but nothing that needs to be fixed." That assessment is only partly right. Hal does not need any more procedures to fix severe blockages, but he still has extensive plaque lining the entire coronary tree. Then how could we measure the volume of plaque lining Hal's arteries?

With present technology, it is impossible to directly measure the volume of plaque in the arteries of a living human being. (We could, of course, do this in an autopsy.) Intracoronary ultrasound provides a pretty good estimation, but it is invasive, expensive, and does carry real risk of complications (like tearing the artery).

Can we quantify volume of plaque easily, non-invasively, precisely, and inexpensively in a living person? Recall our discussion of the various components that make up atherosclerotic plaque. What if *one* of the components of plaque could be measured precisely? What if this component was present in a *consistent proportion* in everyone's plaques? We could then measure a single component and use this indirect measure to *calculate* the total volume of plaque. That is the basic principle behind scoring coronary calcium, and the approach that might have saved Hal's life had he known the extent of plaque he had hidden within.

The beginnings of calcium scoring

While at the Mayo Clinic, Dr. John Rumberger examined the hearts of people who had died (both from heart disease and other causes) and studied both the amount of calcium and the total amount of plaque in their coronary arteries by microscopic examination. He discovered that, regardless of age or sex, calcium comprised 20% of the volume of atherosclerotic plaque. For example, if there were 2 cubic millimeters of calcium, there would be 2 x 5 = 10 cubic millimeters of total plaque volume. Dr. Rumberger therefore concluded that if calcium could be measured, plaque volume could be easily calculated. But measuring calcium and plaque in arteries removed from the body was not possible in walking, talking people. The next step was to reproduce these observations in living people.

Dr. Rumberger possessed the unique insights of a dual background, a doctorate in electrical engineering, as well as medical training as a physician and cardiologist. Along with his study of calcium in human coronary arteries, Dr. Rumberger was also investigating applications of the new (at the time) electron-beam CT scanner invented several years earlier in the San Francisco area by physicist Dr. Douglas Boyd. Dr. Boyd had developed a CT scanner that could obtain images at extremely rapid speed, requiring a small fraction of the time required by other CT scanners. CT scanners in the 1980's required a full 1 to 2 seconds to obtain each cross-sectional image of the body. This may seem fast until you realize how much motion goes on inside the living human body.

The applications of this "ultra-fast" CT scanner, which he subsequently called "electron-beam tomography", or EBT, were not evident at first. Among the first useful applications was in young children, who, as any parent knows, are unable to lie still long enough to obtain images on a conventional CT scanner.

Dr. Boyd envisioned applications in the heart. The slow scan time of other CT devices rendered them useless for imaging the heart. The human heart beats, on average, 70 beats per minute. There are also multiple phases of motion in the heart during each heart beat (atrial systole and diastole; ventricular systole and diastole). Even if you hold your breath (to eliminate motion of the nearby lungs), you have motion in the coronary arteries of two inches per second. That means, if you had a camera trying to obtain still-frame images of the heart with a shutter speed of a full second (1000 milliseconds), you would record a picture that traced (back and forth and rotational) movement of up to two inches in that second. On conventional CT scanners, the heart appears as a meaningless blur, where no detail can be discerned. If you instead had a camera—or a scanner—that could obtain images in fractions of a second, you could eliminate blur-producing movement.

Dr. Rumberger proposed that the unique rapid scanning feature of Dr. Boyd's EBT device could be used to quantify the calcium of coronary arteries. Its split-second scanning time could essentially freeze the motion of a beating heart, exposing even tiny collections of calcium in coronary artery plaque that are commonly a millimeter or so in diameter. When tested in living humans, the EBT scanner, in fact, provided wonderfully detailed images of calcium in the arteries despite the heart's rapid motion. Because precise quantification of calcium could provide an indirect measure of the total plaque volume in a person's coronary arteries, Dr. Rumberger proposed that coronary calcium could provide a "yardstick" of coronary plaque.

Dr. Rumberger initially encountered skepticism from physicians, many of whom were already aware that calcium was a component of atherosclerotic

A coronary artery in cross-section. Plaque is darkly-shaded; white represents calcium in the plaque. If the *area* occupied by calcium were 2.0 mm, then the total plaque area would be 5 x 2.0 = 10.0 mm.

If we examined the entire length of the artery, we would then know the *volume* of plaque present. Knowing the quantity of calcium can therefore provide a method of measuring the volume of coronary plaque.

coronary plaque. This wasn't entirely new information. After all, for years, cardiologists had noticed that patients with the most severe coronary disease (generally elderly patients who came to the hospital with heart attacks or had undergone multiple heart procedures) commonly had calcium in their coronary arteries. The calcium, in fact, was readily visualized during heart catheterization as dense white spots or large streaks. In some patients, there was so much calcium that it could be seen even on a simple chest x-ray. Calcium in the coronary arteries was commonly believed to accompany only the most advanced stages of coronary disease.

Dr. Rumberger proved that, if a sensitive and precise tool like the EBT scanner were used, *calcium could be detected and quantified even in the early phases of coronary disease,* years or decades before it was detectable by other techniques. The more advanced the coronary disease, the more extensive the coronary atherosclerotic plaque, and the more calcium would be measured.

(Subsequent studies showed that the relationship is linear.) Since those early observations, Dr. Rumberger and others have shown that even young people can have calcium that can be detected and scored when other techniques fail to show any calcium or plaque whatsoever.

From confusion to understanding

The history of calcium scoring has had its share of confusion and misperceptions. In the early years, many people were scanned and told that they had coronary calcium present. A heart catheterization or stress test would then be performed, and the patient advised, "Your arteries only have mild plaque and your stress test is normal. The heart scan must be wrong." The calcium score was *not* wrong, it just identified plaque at an earlier stage, years before a stress test became abnormal, and years before a severe blockage was present. These doctors often failed to recognize that the mere presence of plaque was a significant risk for heart attack, regardless of whether severe blockage was present or not.

Many critics still cling to the notion that calcium represents advanced disease, not recognizing that improved methods of imaging can detect calcium and therefore coronary plaque during earlier phases of the process. They argue that the deposition of calcium is a phenomenon of aging and has no value in predicting heart attack. But a huge quantity of evidence now supports the concept of calcium scoring. Literally hundreds of scientific and clinical studies have been performed. Virtually every study has persuasively shown that *the coronary calcium score is the single most powerful predictor of heart attack available.* (See Appendix A for a more extensive discussion of these studies.)

Because of scanning speed, the EBT and MDCT devices are the preferred methods to obtain a coronary calcium score. The entire process requires several minutes, the scan itself requires approximately 40 seconds. With current technology, no other method can identify silent plaque so easily, safely, and reliably. In chapter 5, we will discuss the nitty-gritty of calcium scoring in more detail.

Other methods to detect early heart disease:

Though imaging technology is advanced rapidly, many methods are not yet ready for mainstream use. There are several alternatives, however, to coronary calcium scoring using EBT or MDCT scanners that are already available. Let's discuss these alternatives and their strengths and weaknesses.

Carotid Ultrasound

Atherosclerosis is a body-wide disease that affects all arteries of the body. That means plaque can develop simultaneously in the heart (coronary arteries), the brain (carotid arteries and cerebral circulation), the abdomen (abdominal aorta and mesenteric arteries), legs (iliac and femoral arteries), etc. Plaque develops in these parts of the body in parallel to the heart, though to varying degrees.

Most people with atherosclerotic disease tend to first show some evidence of disease in their heart, i.e., they have a heart attack, or develop angina, or undergo a cardiac procedure. The other arteries of the body, though also developing plaque, tend to do so more slowly. This is partly due to the larger diameter of other arteries. Compare their relative sizes: coronary arteries generally measure 3–4 mm in diameter; carotid arteries measure 5–8 mm; femoral (thigh) arteries measure 6–9 mm. Less plaque accumulation is, therefore, required in the smaller heart arteries.

Nonetheless, because there is a parallel tendency for various arteries to develop plaque, some physicians have proposed that other arteries be measured in place of the heart. The imaging technique usually used is ultrasound, since it is easy, painless, and can be somewhat quantitative.

In ultrasound (similar to that used for intracoronary ultrasound), images are generated by a high frequency, sound emitting crystal. The data is processed by a computer and converted into images. The best studied technique involves ultrasound imaging of the carotid arteries, in which the device is applied gently to the neck and the carotid arteries (right and left) are examined. Using this technique, a measure called carotid intimal-medial thickness, or the thickness of plaque forming artery layers, is obtained. There have also been studies examining other arteries of the body (particularly the abdominal aorta, iliac, and femoral arteries), but they correlate less well to heart disease than the carotids.

Among the most experienced in this technique is Dr. Howard Hodis of the University of Southern California. His extensive experience does indeed suggest that measuring carotid artery intimal-medial thickness can predict heart attack risk, is correlated to a moderate degree with the extent of coronary plaque, and can be used to track the course of disease, i.e, progression or regression. This technique has been quite popular in the research setting to examine the efficacy of various cholesterol therapies.

Ultrasound is safe, since no radiation is involved. Devices capable of obtaining quality images are also very widely available. Most hospitals and even many cardiologists' offices will have at least one if not several ultrasound units.

Carotid ultrasound is already routinely performed to look for large plaques that pose risk for stroke.

So why isn't carotid ultrasound done more widely for identification of early heart disease?

There are several reasons. One reason is that the relationship of coronary disease to carotid disease is not perfectly parallel. Each artery responds somewhat differently to various influences and so develops at different rates. Carotid plaque, for instance, is very sensitive to blood pressure effects; coronary plaque is much less so. The correlation is around 60 to 80%, meaning that a certain carotid intimal-medial thickness measurement will be around 60–80% accurate in predicting the extent of coronary plaque. It is, after all, an indirect measure. It would be like buying a used car and trying to gauge the accuracy of the odometer mileage by looking at the wear on the rubber of the gas pedal—you can make relatively crude predictions, but it's not terribly accurate.

Another weakness of carotid ultrasound is the difficulty in using this measure to track plaque behavior in a specific individual. Over a year or two, the change in the carotid intimal-medial thickness can be tenths or hundredths of a millimeter. In practical life in most ultrasound laboratories, this sort of precision is simply not obtainable.

Patients and physicians also struggle to understand this indirect measure. How can scanning a neck artery predict heart attack? That combined with the above technical limitations make this a less attractive choice for use in your prevention program. If EBT or MDCT scans are not available in your area, and a conversation with your physician suggests that someone with expertise with the ultrasound approach is available, only then might carotid ultrasound be a viable alternative for you.

Ankle-Brachial Index

The ankle-brachial index, or ABI, is mentioned just for information. It is not a desirable method of heart disease detection because of some serious shortcomings. Nonetheless, some physicians do recommend this technique to identify people at risk for heart attack.

Just as plaque accumulates in coronary arteries, it can also grow in leg arteries. If sufficiently advanced, blockages reduce blood flow to the legs, even without symptoms. (Blockages in the leg arteries can cause a cramping in the calves, thighs, or buttocks, and is called claudication.) In contrast, the arteries to the arm rarely develop blockages. Some physicians have therefore proposed that, if you compare the blood pressure (an indirect measure of the volume of blood flow) in the legs to that in the arms, it can tell whether you have plaque in the leg arteries. Because atherosclerosis is a body wide disease, if there is plaque in your leg arteries, you likely also have it in your heart's coronary arteries. The ankle-brachial index is simply the ratio of systolic blood pressure in the legs divided by the systolic blood pressure in the arms. If this ratio is <0.9, this indicates that blood flow to the legs is diminished.

The advantage of this test is that it can be done virtually anywhere a blood pressure device is available. Several studies have confirmed that people with low ABI's do indeed have higher risk for heart attack.

There are several critical disadvantages to this test. For one, it is a crude measure of blood flow to the legs, not the heart, and is therefore an indirect measure. The ABI also tends to be a measure of very *advanced* vascular disease. Blood flow is affected only when there is thick plaque lining the entire arterial tree of the legs and severe blockage is present. Just as with stress testing, the great majority of people who have silent heart disease will have *normal* ABI's and it is, therefore, not an effective method to detect early heart disease. Even in people who've had heart attacks or bypass surgery, only about a third will have an abnormal ABI.

ABI is a method of last resort. Choose this approach only if you live in Timbuktu and no better method is available to you and your doctor.

Magnetic Resonance Imaging (MRI)

Various tissues in the body respond differently when placed in a magnetic field. This principle can be applied in an ingenious imaging method called magnetic resonance imaging, or MRI. MRI is already used in mainstream medical practice to image the chest, abdomen, brain, joints, and other organs, with exquisite detail.

One fascinating aspect of MRI is its capacity for tissue characterization, or distinguishing different types of tissues, such as soft and fatty vs. hard and fibrous. Dr. Valentin Fuster and colleagues at the Mt. Sinai School of Medicine have used MRI to image the aorta (the large artery that emerges from the top of the heart and supplies the major branch arteries to the rest of the body). When aortic plaque is imaged before and after cholesterol lowering therapy (statin drugs), the size of the plaque shrinks within a year's time. Previously fatty tissue is also replaced by denser fibrous tissue, suggesting plaque stabilization with diminished tendency to rupture.

The drawback to MRI is that the current devices are too slow to reliably image the rapidly moving coronary arteries. Preliminary efforts have yielded snapshots of portions of the arteries, but imaging the entire coronary tree remains elusive. MRI promises to be an exciting technique to screen people for hidden coronary plaque, but right now it's just too unreliable and not good enough to **Track Your Plaque.**

In chapter 5, we will discuss everything you need to know about the exciting EBT and MDCT technologies that provide coronary plaque measurement in the here-and-now.

Summary

Imaging technologies are advancing at breakneck speed. The days of invasive procedures to diagnose heart disease are going the way of exploratory abdominal surgery and eight track tapes. The newest CT scanning technologies offer the best balance of precision, ease, cost, and availability for detection of coronary plaque. The perennial problem for imaging the heart has been its rapid motion. The most recent CT scanners are "ultra-fast" and able to provide crystal-clear still-frame images. Two CT devices are the pre-eminent leaders in the race to provide mainstream coronary plaque detection: electron-beam tomography (EBT) and multi-detector CT (MDCT).

Chapter 5

Want to know whether you have heart disease?…Know your score!

Everything you need to know about heart scanning

We finally get down to the nitty-gritty of tracking your plaque in this chapter. To see what it's like getting a coronary calcium score, let's accompany Anna through her experience.

A "walk-through" getting a heart scan

Anna has lived all of her adult life in fear of heart disease. Her father died at age 59 of a heart attack, her mother had urgent bypass surgery at age 62. Other relatives in Anna's close, extended family suffered heart attacks or died of heart disease, all between the ages of 40 and 60. Anna just turned 45 and felt that her clock was ticking. She was also very devoted to her husband and seven-year-old daughter and wished to remain alive and healthy for their sakes. Anna heard about **Track Your Plaque** *and asked whether she'd be appropriate for the program, given her family history. I told her she was a* perfect candidate, *and that a heart scan should begin the process.*

Anna called the scanning center and made an appointment. Once at the center, she filled out the basic demographic information on the standard forms (I often tell patients that the paperwork takes longer than the scan!), then was escorted by the technologist, Gail, back to the scanning area. While remaining in her clothes, Anna had EKG leads applied to her chest and she lay down on the scanning table. The technologist, now at the control console behind a glass panel, asked Anna to hold her breath and a several second preliminary scan was performed to identify landmarks in Anna's chest. Anna was then instructed to hold her breath again, this time for 40 seconds, while Anna's heart was scanned. Anna felt the table move slightly beneath her during the scanning process, but little more. A minute later, Anna hopped off the table and the technologist invited Anna to have a seat at the workstation while they reviewed images of her heart.

Who should be scanned?

How do you decide whether you should have a heart scan in the first place?

Many authorities recommend that men over age 40, women over age 45 be scanned and therefore have their heart disease identified and scored. Several studies have demonstrated that, beyond age, there are no safe criteria to reliably decide who should and who shouldn't be scanned. For example, if you scan only people with high LDL cholesterol (e.g., >130 mg/dl), *half the people with heart disease will be missed* and will not be scanned. Likewise, if you scan people with low HDL(<40 mg/dl), you will again miss about half the people with heart disease. Similar patterns apply for any other screening parameter you can devise. No matter what criterion you choose, you will miss a substantial number of people with silent heart disease.

Think about this. Can we screen you for the presence of heart disease by screening you with another test first? You may begin to see the absurdity in this approach. A study by Drs. Arad and Guerci at the St. Francis Medical Center in New York, for instance, showed that 67% of people classified by the widely used Framingham risk scoring system were mis-classified: people labeled low-risk were actually high-risk; people labeled high-risk were actually low-risk.

The likelihood of having silent coronary plaque does correlate well with age, however. The older you are, the more likely you are to have coronary plaque. Using age, significant numbers of men begin to show coronary plaque by heart scanning at age 40 and over; women begin to show plaque over the age of 45. Since *cholesterol values and conventional risk factors cannot be reliably used to decide whether or not to have a scan,* we therefore resort to age as our guide.

If there is some high risk measure in your life (father or grandfather with heart attack before age 55; mother or grandmother before age 65; diabetes, cholesterol >300, HDL<30, smoking), then you might consider being scanned five years earlier than generally recommended (i.e., age 35 for men, 40 for women.) Using age as our criterion provides the best balance between identifying the greatest number of people with hidden heart disease while not subjecting others to unnecessary scans.

Gail pointed out some of the basic anatomical features on Anna's images, like her lungs, spine, the aorta, as well as heart structures. She also showed Anna the small, dense spots colored white within the coronary arteries of the heart, which

Anna observed were present on about five of the 40 cross-sectional images. But Gail advised Anna that, as the technologist performing the scan, she was not qualified to provide Anna with her final score. This would be done later when Anna's scans were reviewed in detail by one of the center's cardiologists.

Later that evening, I reviewed Anna's scans. (I am one of six cardiologists at our center that review patient scans.) Using the computer software that helps calculate the amount of coronary calcium present, I obtained a score of 63. I called Anna at home the next day. I told Anna that a score of 63 in a 45 year old woman was high and confirmed that coronary disease was established and measurable. Based on her score, Anna's near-term risk heart attack was 4.5% per year, a figure that provided Anna some comfort, since she had assumed that it was much higher. But I also pointed out that a 4.5% annual risk represented a 45% likelihood over the next 10 years, at which time Anna would be a relatively young 55 years old. I also pointed out to Anna that her score of 63 would increase at a rate of 30% per year. Do the math: 63, 82, 106, 138, 179, 233, etc. If we permitted Anna's score to increase (as it undoubtedly would without appropriate action), the likelihood of heart attack would rapidly escalate. My message: let's take this score seriously and apply a program of prevention. So I advised Anna of the next step in the program.

For Anna, getting a score was easy and painless and, despite her high score for a young woman, actually provided an understandable number to her fears. It made it more real, but also made it seem manageable. Knowing her score also solidified Anna's commitment to beginning a more serious effort at prevention.

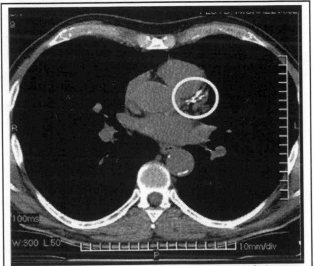

One example image of the 30-40 total images from a heart scan, in this case generated by an EBT scanner. The coronary calcium is circled in white. This is scored (using area and density criteria) and the score of each image added to those of all other images to obtain a *total* calcium score.

How much blockage do I have?

Though your score doesn't tell you whether there is a severe blockage, the higher your score the more likely a severe blockage is present. Here's a breakdown:

Score	Amount of plaque present, likelihood of blockage
0	None. Severe blockage highly unlikely.
1-10	Minimal plaque. Severe blockage highly unlikely.
11-100	Mild quantity of plaque. Very low likelihood of severe blockage.
101-400	Moderate quantity of plaque; 11-25% likelihood of severe blockage.
>400	Extensive plaque with >50% likelihood of severe blockage.

At a score of 200, for example, there is an 11-25% chance that a severe blockage is present. A specific calcium score cannot, however, be equated to a specific percent blockage, as plaque accumulates in various patterns. It does not necessarily all accumulate at one spot and thereby create a single severe blockage. The calcium score can only be associated with the *statistical likelihood* of a severe blockage. Recall that we are interested in more than severe blockages. Any amount of plaque, even in the absence of severe blockage, can result in heart attack because of plaque rupture. The more plaque you have along the length of the artery, the greater the likelihood of plaque rupture.

To predict your heart attack risk, i.e., the likelihood of plaque rupture, we use a measure called "percentile rank." (See below.) Age and sex play a large role in determining how much potential there is for plaque rupture. The younger you are, the more likely a specific quantity of plaque will cause heart attack; the older you are, the less potential there is for the same quantity of plaque to cause heart attack. Percentile rank incorporates age in considering your calcium score. In addition, because women can be at risk for trouble at lower scores for men, we need to compare women to women and men to men. For instance, a calcium score of 90 in a 75 year old man presents low risk for heart attack (This score would be in the 25th percentile.) The very same score of 90 in a 48 year old woman (greater than 90th percentile), in contrast, presents a *very high* risk for heart attack. The same amount of plaque is present in both people, but two very different risks are present. Both age and sex are reflected in the percentile rank, which is a better measure of heart attack, or plaque rupture, potential.

What exactly is a calcium "score"?

Anna's score was 63. This might be a great golf score, but what exactly does this "score" represent in the heart?

A heart scan is 30–40 cross-sectional images (each three millimeters thick) of the heart from top to bottom. (The scans overlap in order to not miss any segment of the heart.) Just as I reviewed Anna's scans, a cardiologist (sometimes a radiologist) will review each "slice" and select what he/she believes represents calcified plaque in the coronary arteries. This is a simple, straightforward process, since calcium is easy to distinguish from the surrounding soft heart tissues. A computer decides whether the selected area meets specific density and size criteria. We multiply the area (in square millimeters) by the density of the plaque, and this yields a score for this specific plaque. Then we score all the plaques in every image slice and add all the scores up. This yields a *total* score, the one reported to the patient (the number 63 reported to Anna). You will sometimes hear the total score called an "Agatston" score, named after Dr. Arthur Agatston from Miami, who first developed this method of adding up and comparing scores from different people. Dr. Agatston's method is now one of the standard calculations performed on all heart scans.

Remember: the higher your score, the more plaque lines your coronary arteries.

Does the calcium score predict heart attack in your future?

No test, no matter how good, can serve perfectly as a crystal ball, but your heart scan score can still do a pretty darn good job of predicting your heart disease future.

In most centers, your total calcium score is compared with a database of 35,000 other people who've also been scanned, based on the enormous experience accumulated by Dr. George Kondos at the University of Illinois–Chicago. Using Dr. Kondos' database, we can compare your score with that of other people your age and sex. We report this as your "percentile rank". The percentile rank is probably the best predictor of heart attack risk we have, probably even better than your score alone. For example, Anna's score of 63, when compared to other women the same age, provided a percentile rank of 90%. This means that 90% of all women her age had lower scores, 10% of women her age had higher scores. The 90th percentile also tells us that Anna's risk for heart attack is 4.5% per year (see table).

The percentile rank provides insight into the aggressiveness of plaque growth. Dr. Paolo Raggi of Tulane University in New Orleans, Louisiana, has extensively researched this phenomenon. Dr. Raggi was the first to observe that the same score in different age groups and sexes predict different risks for heart attack. For instance, a score of 100 in a 48-year-old man represents a small to moderate amount of plaque. It reflects moderately aggressive plaque growth and moderate risk for heart attack. The identical score of 100 in a 65 year-old man represents the exact same amount of plaque that is not as active since it took 65 years to accumulate, rather than 48, and poses only *small* risk for heart attack. The same score of 100 in a 48 year-old woman, however, represents the same amount of plaque but reflects aggressive plaque growth and *high* risk for heart attack. The same heart scan score can, therefore, mean very different things, depending on age and sex. We resort to percentile rank to better predict risk for heart attack.

Calcium score "red flags" for danger

Are there calcium scores that can be "red flags" for potential danger in the near-future?

There definitely are, and these red flags are generally any score in the *90th percentile or greater*. However, even if the scanning center you choose does not report a percentile rank, here are some general guidelines for identifying red flags:

- If you are younger than 55 years old, a score >100
- If you are 55 years old or older, a score >200
- Score >1000. This is the most dangerous of all.

These are scores that may present dangers even in the next few months. Prompt action on your part is warranted. Discuss your score with your physician so that you can talk about intensified prevention, the need for stress testing, and additional testing, if necessary.

Percentile rank and annual risk for heart attack

Heart scans are generally reported as both a score and a percentile rank. The percentile rank is the best predictor of the future risk of heart attack.

Percentile Rank	Annual Heart Attack risk (% per year)
<25%	< 1%
25-50%	1-2 %
50-75%	2-3%
75-90%	3-4%
>90%	>4.5%

Don't be misled by the seemingly small risk of heart attack per year: Multiply any of the annual rates of risk by 10 to approximate your 10 year risk. For example, if you are in the 50-75th percentile group, your one year risk of heart attack is only 2-3%. But over a 10 year period it is 20-30%-a high-risk by anyone's measure.

For physicians and readers interested in a more thorough scientific discussion of the data behind the calcium scoring, please see Appendix A at the back of this book.

Do I need bypass surgery?

People often ask, "If I have a high score, do I need bypass surgery?"

Just having plaque in your coronary arteries does not necessarily mean that you need to have bypass surgery or other major procedures. There are additional evaluations that may need to be done to help you and your doctor make this determination (discussed later). *In the absence of symptoms*, just having plaque detectable by scoring should rarely—perhaps *never*—be the sole indication for a major procedure. In other words, just having plaque measured by a calcium score, even high scores, does not necessarily mean your arteries need to be bypassed or stented.

That said, it is true that the higher your score, the more likely it is that your coronary plaque is so extensive that a major procedure may be necessary for your safety. In our center, approximately 30% of all people with scores exceeding 1000 (very high!) undergo hospital procedures like heart catheterization, angioplasty and stent placement, and bypass surgery. However, this decision can almost *never* be made on the basis of your heart scan score alone.

Despite the pitfalls of stress testing to detect hidden plaque, this is an instance where a stress test can help. (See box, "Do I need a stress test?") A stress test (usually with imaging, such as thallium) can show whether your plaque blocks blood flow to various regions of the heart muscle. It can also indicate whether physical activity generates any dangerous responses. If you are without symptoms and have a normal stress test, it is rare that hospital procedures will be required.

Calcium scoring technologies—an evolving field

Can you just go to your neighborhood hospital and get a heart scan on their CT device? After all, nearly all major hospitals have at least one CT scan device in their radiology departments.

In general, you cannot. Or, perhaps, I should say you *should* not. As we discussed earlier in the book, hospitals just are not in the business of preventing heart disease and have, therefore, not invested in technology that is useful for these purposes. The CT scanners in the majority of hospitals, though similar, are different devices in several critical ways.

First of all, heart scanning demands speed. Dr. Rumberger originally chose the EBT scanner years ago because of its ability to obtain split-second scans. Most CT scanners in the hospital (which are perfectly suitable for other purposes, like imaging stationary organs such as the brain or liver) require 500–1000 msec (0.5–1.0 sec) for each image, *up to 10 times slower* than the EBT scanner. For this reason, CT scans obtained in most hospitals will show the heart as a large blur, since the heart moves about two inches during that time. Rapidly moving, small calcified plaques in the coronary arteries, often measuring a millimeter in diameter, simply cannot be reliably imaged with these devices.

The so-called spiral or helical CT scanners, named because of the rotating arm, or gantry, of the scanner that spins around the body of the patient, have improved on the slow scanning of the older machines. But this heavy rotating gantry can only move so fast, and scans obtained with these devices generally scan at an effective speed of around 500 msec (0.5 sec), still too slow for reliable heart imaging.

New techniques to circumvent the physical limitations of scan speed have led to the development of a new generation of scanners called

Do I need a stress test?

If you have a calcium score >0, do you need a stress test? This is a common question from patients as well as doctors. Here are practical guidelines for people *without symptoms* (no chest pains, breathlessness, etc.). The presence of *symptoms* suggestive of heart disease can be a reasonable indication to perform a stress test, *regardless of the score*, low or high. This should be decided by your doctor.

If your score is:	Likelihood of abnormal stress test
0-10	<1%
11-100	2-3%
101-400	11-12%
>400	>50%

This provides a good starting point for thinking about the need for a stress test (thallium or equivalent). If, for instance, your calcium score is 25, the likelihood of an abnormal stress test is only 2-3%, and any area of poor blood flow detected will likely be very small. Most physicians and patients would therefore choose not to proceed to stress testing, provided you are without symptoms. On the other hand, scores of >400 should nearly always prompt additional evaluation like stress testing. Some of these people may require "revascularization", or some means of restoring the inadequate flow identified by stress tests.

If some people need to have a stress test anyway, why bother with the calcium score? *Because the majority of people (>90%) of people with coronary plaque will have normal stress tests.* Any quantity of coronary plaque-whether or not it yields a stress test abnormality-poses risk for heart attack. Even people with a score of 400, a high score signifying advanced and extensive plaque, only have a 50% chance of having it detected by stress testing. The other 50% with normal stress tests would be told their coronaries were fine, even though they're really loaded with plaque.

A word of warning: beware of the uninformed doctor who, when presented with your coronary calcium score, says something like, "I don't know what this stupid test means. I didn't order it. If you really want to know if you have blockage, just have a heart catheterization." There are reasonable indications for heart catheterization (like progressive or disabling symptoms of heart disease, a large area of poor blood flow to the heart, abnormal weakness of the heart muscle, or life-threatening rhythm disturbances), but finding out if you have coronary plaque in the absence of symptoms and without a stress test is *not* among them.

"multi-detector" spiral or helical scanners. Multi-detector scanners also use a rotating gantry. But instead of trying to rotate the gantry faster, engineers have designed these scanners with more than one detector ring that capture x-ray beams after passing through the body. The newest generation of scanners have 4, 8, 16, and even 32 detector rings. This multiple ring approach has shortened the effective scan time down to about 250 msec (0.25 sec), getting close to the 100 msec of the EBT scanner.

Is 250 msec. obtainable on the most advanced multi-detector device close enough to the 100 msec gold standard? Experience suggests it's pretty good. The existing data also confirm that scores obtained on both devices are comparable. A score of 200, say, on an EBT device, will also likely be around 200 on a multi-detector device.

Do I need a heart catheterization?

Too often, an elevated calcium score leads to cardiac catheterization, an invasive procedure to inject x-ray dye into your arteries that identifies the "need" for stents or bypass surgery. Does having a high calcium score mean you automatically need heart catheterization?

Absolutely not. The need for catheterization should generally be decided on the basis of symptoms and/or the findings on stress testing. Even though your calcium score identifies the presence of plaque, having plaque by itself is almost *never* a reason to have heart catheterization or other invasive procedures.

Measuring coronary plaque is one of the breakthrough technologies available today that will have significant impact on reducing the numbers of people dying of heart disease or having to undergo major heart procedures. Unfortunately, many physicians who simply do not understand the technology advise patients that having an elevated calcium score means they need major cardiac procedures. Should you receive advice like this, you should run, not walk, to get a second opinion. Let me state this again: *The presence of coronary plaque detected by EBT or MDCT scanning by itself rarely mandates the performance of major cardiac procedures in the absence of symptoms and with a negative stress test.* The need for major cardiac procedures like heart catheterization, which then often leads to stents, bypass surgery, etc., in *asymptomatic* people should be based on the finding of "ischemia", or poor blood flow to one or more territories of the heart, *not* the presence of plaque. Another reasonable indication for proceeding to heart catheterization would be abnormal heart muscle weakness, usually detected by an echocardiogram or physical examination.

If no symptoms are present and there is a calcium score sufficiently high to justify stress testing (see box above, "Do I need a stress test?"), then a stress test should almost always be performed first before considering a heart catheterization. If symptoms are present that your doctor deems suspicious for heart disease, then it may be reasonable to proceed to major procedures without stress testing.

If you have no symptoms and your calcium score is >0, before the need for invasive cardiac procedures is decided, you will need a stress test. The only exception would be if your heart muscle shows abnormal weakness. It's as simple as that. If you're told otherwise, be highly suspicious of the advice.

Another important distinction among the various technologies is the quantity of radiation your body is exposed to when you have a scan. Think of the heart scan as being just like a mammogram: A screening test should be not only reliable and accurate, but should also introduce as little risk as possible. In screening for breast cancer with mammography, for instance, women desire a test that can accurately identify early cancers, but not with such high radiation exposure that the test itself causes cancer. The analogous situation arises with coronary calcium scoring. The test needs to be accurate in detecting early heart disease, but it should be performed with as little radiation as possible and should not add substantially to cancer risk.

The EBT and MDCT scanners remain the preferred devices in this regard, with relatively low levels of radiation exposure. An EBT scan exposes you to radiation equivalent to somewhere between two and four chest x-rays, MDCT scans slightly more. The older helical and spiral devices (single detector ring) vary widely in their radiation exposure, but generally deliver *4 to 20-times greater* radiation—unacceptable levels. If given a choice, an EBT scanner or a four-slice or greater MDCT scanner are the preferred devices to use.

All across the country, scan sites are popping up quickly. (To locate a scanner in your area, see Appendix B.) If you know of a scanner in your area, it is worth a call to the center. Ask the receptionist or technologist at the center what kind of device they're using. If they are unwilling or unable to tell you the type of scanner they're using, consider going elsewhere.

Another word of caution: The excitement for this new technology has also encouraged the appearance of "me too" scanners, many of which are mobile and travel to your town offering scans at cut rates. The same principles regarding image acquisition speed and radiation dose apply. Should you consider having your scan on such a device, please be certain to ask what type of scanner is being used. Unfortunately, many of these mobile, cut-rate services use primitive scanners (so-called "axial" scanners, many of which were manufactured in the early and mid-1990's) which really have no business offering heart scans, due to their unacceptable imprecision in scoring coronary calcium and the high dose of radiation required to imitate a true heart scan.

The EBT and MDCT heart scanners therefore represent the "top of the heap." They provide the easiest, safest, and most accurate method available to quantify atherosclerotic coronary plaque.

Keeping score of your heart disease

Just as you keep score during a baseball game, you can do the same with your coronary plaque.

Let me tell you about Stephen's experience.

Stephen, a 57-year-old businessman, had a heart scan two years earlier at age 55, mostly because his wife "made him do it." Stephen's score: 227, in the 75th percentile for men his age. When Stephen told his doctor about the scan and showed him the report, the doctor looked at it for a moment, then handed it back to him and said, "I don't know what the heck this means. This isn't even a real test. We'll do a stress test."

Well, Stephen's stress test was normal and the doctor declared the heart scan useless and a waste of money. He told Stephen to go about his life and return in a year.

But Stephen's wife, Laura, knew better. She'd asked numerous questions during her scan and recognized that there was valuable information in the heart scan score. She had a hard time persuading Stephen to share her views at first, given the doctor's negative comments. A year later, Laura managed to convince Stephen to undergo another heart scan. His score: 363—a 60% increase. This really grabbed Stephen's attention. He didn't bother telling his doctor but came to my office instead. When I told him that his increasing score put him at very high risk for heart attack despite the normal stress test, he agreed to participate in the program without hesitation in the hopes of averting catastrophe.

If, like Stephen, nothing is done about the causes of your plaque, your score can increase 30%, 40%, or more per year. Your score can be used not only as a yardstick for the initial measurement of coronary plaque, but it can also be used to track its increase or decrease over time. People who experience this rate of increase launch themselves into a very high risk group for future heart attack, as much as *20-fold higher* than people with unchanging scores. Stephen (and his doctor) allowed his score to increase to 363, increasing his risk 20-fold, as compared to his score at the initial 227.

People who succeed in halting their score don't have zero percent risk of heart attack (*nobody* has a zero risk), but the risk becomes low. Scores that fall *below* the starting value (i.e., shrinking plaque) indicate even lower and lower risk of heart attack. *Achieving a stable or decreasing heart scan score can therefore be an important goal to sharply reduce your risk of heart attack.*

When considering a repeat scan, you should do so no sooner than a year after the first. Even better, your second scan should be timed approximately one year after the lipid/lipoprotein abnormalities causing your plaque are corrected.

Correction of the lipid/lipoprotein patterns that caused your heart disease can require several months. Repeating your heart scan a year after lipids/lipoproteins are corrected will give you an idea of what impact you've had on your score in light of your corrected patterns. In our center, experience has shown that most people require a full year or more to halt an increasing score, or achieve a decrease. This is discussed further in the next chapter.

What if you've already had a heart procedure?

Some unique approaches are required if you've had coronary stent(s) or bypass surgery.

Coronary stents are a fine tubular mesh constructed of stainless steel or similar material. Metal looks just like calcium when visualized by any CT scan device. Even though the structure of a stent can be distinguished, it cannot be reliably differentiated from calcium that the stent(s) covers. For this reason, if you have one or more stents in a single coronary artery, you can still obtain a score, but the score will not include the stented artery. The total score will therefore underestimate the full extent of coronary plaque and will distort the percentile rank, making it inaccurate. Nonetheless, you can still track your score on future scans when the same two arteries are scored. So having a single artery with stent(s) still permits you to obtain a useful score.

The real problem is people with multiple arteries (two or three) that are stented. The stented arteries can no longer be excluded without sacrificing crucial information. We are presently researching methods to circumvent this limitation, but at present, the presence of multiple arteries with stents is a real stumbling block. People with this problem can still obtain great benefit from many of the other concepts in **Track Your Plaque**, but the scoring process is one step that is impossible with present technology.

The other problem area is people who have had bypass surgery. When the surgeon places a bypass graft, your own coronary arteries are distorted by the act of manual handling. In addition, bypass grafts themselves often obscure the images of your own arteries, making the scoring process difficult or impossible. Having bypass grafts might not entirely eliminate the possibility of obtaining a usable calcium score, but in our center less than half the people with prior bypass surgery can be scored. Usually the only way to find out if you can get a score is to give it a try, provided the center you use has an interpreting physician willing to devote the effort. People with bypass surgery can still obtain great benefit from the other **Track Your Plaque** concepts, minus the scoring component.

What does a heart scan cost? What about insurance coverage?

As the number of scanners capable of performing coronary calcium scoring grows, the price of getting a scan has plummeted. In many cities, you can get a heart scan for $200 or less. Though this may seem a lot at first, compare this to the cost of a very similar (often lower quality) CT scan of the chest performed in a hospital. Price? Around $4000! Heart scans are a bargain.

Just because a test provides valuable information doesn't mean your insurance will cover it. Insurance coverage for EBT or MDCT scans is variable, depending on the state you live in and other factors generally beyond your control. You may encounter a wide range of responses from your insurance company from outright silly comments like "We don't cover experimental procedures" (it's *not* experimental, of course), or you may be fully covered. It helps to ask ahead of time. It also helps to have a doctor's order for a scan. This sometimes is a factor in your insurer's decision. (Some states require a physician's order to obtain a scan, while other states will permit you to undergo a scan without a physician's order. Just ask the scanning center you're planning to use.) Some employers have special arrangements for their employees to receive a scan at a discount. Even if your company does not have such a program, many employers who've suffered the loss of an employee or borne the extraordinary health insurance expense of employees with heart disease will be receptive to making some kind of contribution.

Many people ask, "If heart scanning prevents heart attacks and expensive heart procedures, why won't health insurers cover it?" First of all, from an insurance perspective, prevention of disease can be very expensive. You may need to treat 20, 30, maybe 50 people to prevent a single heart attack over a two or three-year timeline. Even if prevention of the disease costs only a tenth of the cost of catastrophic care, e.g., bypass surgery, the greater number of people treated to prevent the process can erode any savings. Secondly, most people will change insurance companies every two to three years. Why would company X spend money to prevent a heart attack and expensive procedures 10 years from now when you will likely be insured by company Y by that time? It makes no financial sense from the perspective of your insurance company to prevent your heart attack, even if we knew for certain it would occur in, say, 7 or 8 years.

Even if insurance does not cover the cost of a heart scan, it is money well spent for the priceless information it provides. For the cost of a new DVD player or dinner for four, you can obtain high-tech insight into your heart health that just might save your life.

In the next chapter, we discuss the concept of score reduction in more detail and why this can be such an important goal.

Summary

Getting your coronary calcium score with an EBT or MDCT scanner is Step 1 in your personal **Track Your Plaque** program. These technologies offer a safe, convenient, and inexpensive method of quantifying plaque in the coronary arteries. The calcium score provided by these tests gives you an indirect though extremely reliable gauge of the plaque present in your coronary arteries. The higher your score, the greater the quantity of plaque in your coronary arteries, and the higher the risk for heart attack and other cardiac catastrophes. The coronary calcium score can be used as a yardstick for plaque and can be tracked for its increase, stabilization, or decrease.

Chapter 6

Can I reduce my heart scan score?

*If we can accurately measure coronary plaque,
we should aim to reduce it.*

Like a weed in your garden, coronary plaque grows rapidly. With growth unchecked, plaque scores increase, on average, at a rate of 30–35% per year. A starting score of 100 will become 130, 169, 220, 286, 371,…kaboom!!!

Heart attack doesn't necessarily occur once you exceed a specific value, but the likelihood of heart attack escalates dramatically along with your score. It's like building a house of cards: the more cards you stack, the shakier the structure, until you add that final card and it all collapses. *Growing* plaque is *unstable* plaque.

If you know your heart scan score, your future is at a crossroads. One path leads to life with a score that doesn't increase (or decreases) versus another path with your score increasing the expected 30% per year. How different is your future between the two paths? Even in the ensuing two years, an increasing score means your heart attack risk skyrockets *20-fold*. It means you're getting closer and closer to that day when catastrophe strikes. In contrast, a stable or decreasing score means high likelihood of remaining free of heart attack and major heart procedures. There is tremendous benefit to stopping your score.

Can you reduce your score? Most people can, given the proper tools, adherence to the program, and sufficient time.

What does it mean to reduce my score?

When your heart scan score is held stable or is reduced, this is evidence that not only is your plaque no longer growing, but it is being inactivated. (Plaque activity cannot be directly measured in a live human, so we need to rely on indirect methods.) You have re-absorbed the cholesterol in the plaque, shrunk plaque size, turned off inflammatory processes and enzymes, and extracted some of the calcium. When plaque is inactivated, it is far less likely to rupture and cause heart attack.

You and I can live happily with our plaque. We just don't want growing and potentially rupture-prone plaque. A stable or reduced heart scan score can be viewed as a surrogate, or indirect, measure of plaque inactivation. Inactive plaque is far less likely to rupture, to cause heart attack and other catastrophes.

How do I know if my score has increased or decreased?

How do you know what your plaque is doing, shrinking or growing? Simple: get another scan.

Many people ask: Doesn't having a "perfect" cholesterol value with treatment (e.g., a statin drug) guarantee a reduction in score? Unfortunately, it does not. How about a perfect lifestyle—strict adherence to diet, vigorous exercise, adequate sleep, etc? This won't guarantee that plaque shrinks, either. Cholesterol values, even lipoproteins (discussed in chapter 7) are only starting points to identify potential tools to shrink your plaque. The only way to measure results in a specific individual is to re-measure the quantity of plaque present—get another scan. Lowering cholesterol, eating healthy, etc. are indeed helpful and enhance the likelihood of stopping your score, but no specific measure guarantees it.

In fact, there is *nothing* that truly tells you what your score is doing except...another score. Tracking your plaque is therefore a two scan experience. There is no way to accurately and reliably predict what your score has done without looking at the score again.

In my experience, the majority of people who adhere to **Track Your Plaque** can slow or completely stop the otherwise inevitable increase in score, though the time required to do so may vary. In the first year, if all the proper steps are taken, a very realistic goal is to achieve an increase in score of no more than 10%. The existing data suggest that a score increase of <10% represents low-risk, and heart attack becomes less and less likely as your plaque is inactivated. Rates of increase of 10-20% in score are very common but suggest that your program has room for improvement. I call this a "deceleration" of your score, as it represents a slowing of the expected rate of progression of 30–35% per year. Increases of 10-20% means that plaque is still growing at a rate that still poses some danger, and a re-examination of lipid and lipoprotein endpoints is in order. (See below.)

A zero-percent increase or even a decrease in score is more commonly encountered after two years on this program. Obtaining a reduction of score with present treatments is therefore a one to two-year long process for most participants.

It is important to point out that the lower your starting score, the more easily it is reduced. Scores of 200 or less have a much greater chance of being lowered in the first year than scores >200. In our program, 75% of people with starting scores of <200 succeed in the first year. This drops to 30% success in the first year if your score is >200, 50% by end of year 2. The message here is clear: the earlier you start to Track Your Plaque, the more control you will have over your heart's future. Nonetheless, if you start with a higher score, don't give up hope. You will just have to work harder and be patient, since this process requires at least two years for most people to enjoy substantial score-reducing or slowing effects.

Certain groups of people can anticipate greater difficulty in controlling their score. People with established diabetes will especially struggle. Unfortunately, if you've already been diagnosed with diabetes, reducing your score is unlikely. The Track Your Plaque principles still do represent the most powerful prevention program you can follow, but it is more likely that you simply "decelerate" your plaque growth with these efforts, rather than achieve score reduction as long as you remain diabetic.

People with the metabolic syndrome (see chapter 8) who have a combination of low HDL, high triglycerides, high blood pressure, blood sugar levels >110, and are often overweight, will also struggle to control their plaque. The metabolic syndrome generally precedes the onset of full-blown diabetes but has a similar, though lesser, impact on plaque. The most powerful tool for control of plaque growth for many people like this is weight-loss. (Discussed further in chapter 10.) It is possible to control plaque with metabolic syndrome in the picture, but it can be considerably more difficult.

Once score stabilization or reduction is achieved, the need for any future scans to detect additional change is really an individual decision. Since the score has started to drop, the most important goal has been achieved. It is worth considering another scan, however, if there is some significant change in your program. For instance, significant weight gain, development of diabetes, or a prolonged period of treatment interruption are among reasons for repeating a scan despite initial control of the score.

What does a zero percent change or a reduction in heart scan score mean? A zero-percent change means your plaque is no longer growing at the alarming rate of 30–35% per year. A reduction in score signifies actual shrinkage of coronary plaque. Both situations suggest that dangerous characteristics of plaque (inflammation and erosion of the structural tissues) are being turned-off. It also means that, although plaque is still present, the fatty portion of plaque is being replaced by solid structural tissues that allow plaque to exist quietly without inflammation and without the active processes that cause rupture. A decreasing heart scan score provides powerful indirect evidence that your plaque is becoming stable and inactive.

What if my score *doesn't* stop going up?

What if your score fails to stabilize and continues to increase, even after two years of effort? Does this mean heart attack is inevitable? Should you just throw up your hands and schedule your hospitalization?

No, of course not. But it is worth taking this increase very seriously. In the absence of symptoms, you and your doctor may need to repeat your lipoprotein analysis to be certain you are achieving the desired endpoints. If you are not at the recommended endpoints (discussed in chapter 8), changes in your program will be necessary to achieve or maybe even exceed endpoints. You should also re-examine your lifestyle changes of diet and exercise (detailed in the next several chapters). A lax approach to plain old diet and exercise are common reasons for imperfect control of plaque.

If you've started with conventional lipid analysis rather than lipoproteins, you and your doctor should consider obtaining the more comprehensive and powerful lipoprotein analysis to identify hidden deficiencies in your program. Usually, your score will fall in line with some additional tweaking of your program.

Is there a rate of increase in score—say 10 or 15% in a year—that is "safe"? Is there some degree of score increase that can occur without exposing you to a significant risk of heart attack? Rates of increase of 20% or more per year are clearly high-risk and should prompt a very serious re-examination of your lipoproteins and overall program. Though not as desirable as zero percent change or a drop, a rate of increase of <10% is probably safe within the first year. Rates of 10-20% still pose risk, and suggest room for improvement in your program.

Let's go on to Step 2 of **Track Your Plaque,** in which we focus on identifying the causes of coronary plaque.

Summary

Coronary plaque grows at the alarming rate of 30–35% per year. Being able to measure plaque precisely through coronary calcium scoring provides a means to potentially control the growth of plaque. Tracking your score provides powerful feedback on your ability to halt or even shrink plaque. This opens a whole new age of potential coronary plaque regression.

Track Your Plaque

Step 2

Chapter 7

"My doctor said my cholesterol was fine...*So why did I have a heart attack?!*"

Why cholesterol fails in so many people

Rick, a successful real estate developer, has religiously had his cholesterol values monitored every six months since age 38. The numbers have wavered within a narrow range, with LDL cholesterols that have never exceeded 95. "Excellent, as always", his family doctor declares. But a heart attack struck him down without warning at age 54, leaving him breathless and fatigued, as well as anxious for his future. It caused him to demand, "My doctor said my cholesterol was fine. So why did I have a heart attack?!"

Rick deserves an answer.

The answer is that there are many ways to develop heart disease. The list of potential causes of coronary plaque is long. In fact, *most people with coronary disease have five, six, or more reasons to have plaque.* High cholesterol is just one cause on this list. Yet most of the time your doctor makes a myopic attempt to decide whether you have heart disease by looking only at your cholesterol.

Keep in mind that we will *not* use any of these tests to uncover the presence of hidden plaque. That's the role of the heart scan. Measuring and scoring plaque brings the picture into sharp focus. If you have an abnormal heart scan score (above 0), you *know* that you have coronary plaque. Heart attack may be in your future, and the higher the score, the greater the quantity of hidden plaque, and the greater your future heart attack risk. We don't need risk factor assessment to tell us this.

Who needs cholesterol?

"Now wait a minute!" you might say. "If we use calcium scoring to detect coronary plaque, can't we just throw cholesterol away?"

In a way, that's right. Once your heart scan score shows you have coronary plaque, we no longer need cholesterol to make this initial decision. It doesn't matter whether your cholesterol is 150 or 350. If you have coronary plaque, you have coronary artery disease and potential for heart attack in the future—period. In **Track Your Plaque**, we don't have to use risk factors to tell us who will or who won't have a heart attack. We also won't rely on the calculations intended to improve on single measures, like the "Framingham risk calculator" or the cholesterol/HDL ratio. If you have a calcium score >0 (or if you've had coronary disease identified by some other means like heart attack, angioplasty, stent, or bypass surgery) then and only then can we begin to discuss how plaque got started in the first place. (The only time we use various risk factors to identify future risk of heart attack is when your heart scan score is zero. In other words, perhaps you are 28 years old and your heart attack is still 30 years away. You have no measurable coronary plaque, or, in this case, you're too young to have a scan, but risk factor assessment can still be used as a crude means of anticipating your long-term statistical risk for heart disease. In this situation, risk factors should be taken seriously and treated to standard guidelines, as determined by your doctor.)

So should we completely discard lipid measures like cholesterol, LDL, and HDL? No, absolutely not. Despite their shortcomings, these simple measures still have their usefulness. While they are of limited helpfulness in uncovering hidden heart disease, they are useful to identify some of the *causes* of plaque.

Risk factors are therefore primarily useful as *tools for treatment*. LDL is less a measure of risk, but a more effective tool for management. Even though your LDL cholesterol doesn't tell us whether you do or do not have coronary plaque, lowering it can nonetheless help control plaque. It doesn't end there, however. If treatment of coronary disease were as easy as treating your LDL cholesterol, lowering LDL cholesterol would cure heart disease. It does not. Here is where the idea of lipoprotein analysis shines.

Treating LDL cholesterol does not cure heart disease because there are many other ways to develop heart disease besides LDL. Let's put aside for a moment obvious causes like smoking, hypertension, and diabetes, and focus on causes that are hidden. Sometimes other causes are suggested by the lipid panel (LDL, HDL, triglycerides, the most common combination of tests ordered by doctors), such as low HDL. Other times, the causes are not at all evident in the lipid panel and can only be uncovered through additional testing.

I'll use Lisa's story to illustrate:

Lisa is a 43-year-old wife and mother of two teenage children. She works as a laboratory technologist at a local hospital. Lisa has lived with growing concern over her future because of her father, who suffered a fatal heart attack without warning at age 59. More recently, Lisa's brother, aged 45 (just two years older) had his second heart attack. Thankfully, he survived and had a stent placed in one of his coronary arteries. Lisa was very interested in avoiding heart procedures and in not having a heart attack.

Lisa has an upbeat, pleasant personality. When you meet Lisa, you instantly like her. She is a non-smoker, thin and physically active. At the start of the program, her LDL (bad) cholesterol was 68, HDL (good) cholesterol a very wonderful 74, all without treatment. In fact, her family physician told her that she had escaped the bad genetics shared by her father and brother.

She underwent a heart scan. Her score: 459, in the worst 1% of all women her age (99th percentile). In fact, Lisa had the highest score I've ever seen in a woman less than 50 years old.

Had we confined ourselves to lipid values to decide whether Lisa did or didn't have hidden coronary disease, we would have completely misjudged her. She would have received a pat on the back and been told to stop worrying. In reality, Lisa was at extremely high risk for heart attack. If Lisa's lipid values were better than perfect, where did her heart disease come from? And if we don't know where it came from, how can we hope to keep it from getting worse?

Through a more thorough analysis, Lisa proved to have an inherited abnormality called lipoprotein a, or Lp(a). This, in fact, was the only abnormality in an otherwise perfect profile. Given her heart scan score, Lisa's risk for heart attack over the next decade was 45%, with virtually a 100% chance of heart attack or unstable symptoms sufficient to require bypass surgery or stents over a longer timeline. (By the way, Lisa's stress test was normal. Had we relied on a stress test to tell us whether Lisa was at risk, we again would have completely missed the boat.)

A heart scan succeeded in revealing the true extent of Lisa's heart disease, while standard risk factors failed miserably. Though most people like Lisa have a half dozen reasons for plaque, Lisa was an exception in this regard, having only a single compelling reason. But Lisa is a glaring example of how many of the hidden causes of heart disease are not revealed by standard cholesterol testing.

Let me tell you about Bob:

Bob is a 49-year-old mason who owns a small construction company with his brother, Dave. Bob is slender and muscular due to the demands of his work, laying brick and cinder blocks much of his day. Bob smoked for 15 years, but quit in his early 40s. His family doctor had identified high LDL cholesterols in the 200 range, so Bob had been prescribed simvastatin (Zocor) about three years earlier. I had seen Bob's brother, Dave, who I met after a heart scan showing a moderate quantity of coronary plaque. Bob wanted to learn more about the techniques used in **Track Your Plaque.** *Both brothers were motivated to avoid their dad's fate, a bypass operation in his early 60's, which scarred him with an infected chest incision, chronic leg edema, and a faulty memory.*

Bob underwent a heart scan. Sure enough, his score: 929—very high and in the 99th percentile compared to other men his age. (Annual risk for heart attack 4.5%; 10 year risk 45%.) Bob's score, in fact, exceeded his older brother's score by a wide margin. Bob did complain of some aches and pains in his chest and shoulders that he suspected were due to the muscular strain of his work, but I had Bob undergo a stress thallium anyway to help understand the meaning of his symptoms. The stress test was entirely normal, suggesting that Bob's symptoms were unlikely to be from coronary disease.

But Bob had extensive plaque. Where did it come from? Was his prior high LDL cholesterol and prior smoking sufficient explanation? Would lowering LDL with simvastatin and not smoking be enough to keep his heart scan score from climbing higher?

A more thorough assessment of Bob uncovered six *additional causes for his high score, involving abnormalities of several lipoproteins. Based on these results, I added several treatments to Bob's simvastatin, including counseling on specific changes in his diet to help counteract the effects of some of his lipoprotein patterns. One year later, another heart scan score showed a 12% increase in score, representing a marked deceleration over the expected increase.*

Bob's high score was the result of multiple causes, some genetic, some lifestyle related. A high score like Bob's in a relatively young person, even in a former smoker, is nearly always caused by *multiple* abnormalities.

Why does coronary plaque develop in the first place?

Let's talk for a moment about the causes of coronary artery disease, the various reasons plaque accumulates and leads to heart attack. This may help you understand why lipoproteins and other measures beyond cholesterol more accurately identify causes of coronary plaque and heart attack.

The development of atherosclerotic plaque is a complex, multi-faceted process that begins in childhood. The inciting event probably involves injury to the thin walled inner lining of the artery. Injury can take many forms: high blood pressure, excessive fat intake, nicotine, deposition of cholesterol particles, etc. Cholesterol has been a major focus because it is found in abundance within plaques. This led to the over-simplified assumption that high levels of cholesterol in the blood caused cholesterol to be deposited within the artery wall, forming plaque. As we will discuss later, it is not just a high blood cholesterol level that encourages deposition in plaques, but also the *type* of particle that delivers the cholesterol. This is the rationale for studying lipoproteins, the blood protein particles that carry cholesterol and other fats.

Plaques are hotbeds of internal activity. They produce proteins that attract inflammatory white blood cells (called monocytes and macrophages) that infiltrate the plaque, much as they would any wound. Inflammatory cells produce digestive enzymes that weaken plaque structure. The enzymes inadvertently degrade the covering cap of the plaque that separates plaque contents from blood. The cap is then weakened and can rupture, exposing the normally covered plaque contents to blood. This is a highly blood clot promoting situation and is the cause for heart attack in most instances. Plaque inflammation is a hot area for research. One way to indirectly assess the contribution of inflammation to dangerous plaque activity is the measurement of C-reactive protein, or CRP, in the blood.

As plaque grows, small bits of calcium are formed, sometimes as little pebbles and sometimes as larger arcs. This, of course, is the basis for calcium measurement to indirectly measure plaque volume. The larger the plaque grows, the more calcium accumulates (occupying 20% of total plaque volume), the higher your score. The reason why calcium is deposited in the first place, however, is not clear.

Circulating HDL (good) cholesterol particles in the blood are responsible for a process called reverse cholesterol transport, in which HDL particles extract cholesterol from plaque for disposal in the liver. HDL particles are therefore crucial participants in the process of plaque regression. For **Track Your Plaque**, HDL becomes a very important tool. In fact, HDL is one of the most important parameters to measure and correct.

Because blood clot formation is required to suffer a heart attack, people who are prone to blood clotting are at higher risk for heart attack once a plaque ruptures. This is the reason for measuring clotting proteins like fibrinogen. It is also the basis for the reduction in heart attacks provided by aspirin and fish oil, both of which inhibit the clotting of blood platelets.

To date, there are approximately 300 known risk factors that contribute to plaque formation and blood clotting. It becomes impractical to try and correct each and every one of these risk factors. Fortunately, many therapies tend to improve multiple causes. One great example is fish oil, a source of omega-3 fatty acids. Fish oil is a simple, inexpensive preparation that lowers triglycerides, lowers fibrinogen, has anti-inflammatory activity, reduces the stickiness of inflammatory cells to the plaque wall, reduces post-prandial (after meals) blood fat levels, and can reduce the risk of death from coronary disease by stabilizing the heart's potential for unstable rhythms. One treatment, multiple benefits.

Lipids and Lipoproteins

When your doctor says your cholesterol is high, what exactly does that mean?

Cholesterol is an *oil-based* substance; blood (actually plasma, the clear fluid that remains when red blood cells are removed) is a *water-based* liquid. Cholesterol does not float freely in your blood. If it did, it would separate just like oil and vinegar. This, of course, does not occur in your blood stream. (You would die if it did.) Cholesterol travels in the blood as a "passenger" on a family of protein particles, called lipoproteins (meaning lipid carrying proteins.) This allows cholesterol to be soluble in blood. It also permits proteins to steer the lipoprotein particle to target the liver, plaque, or other places in the body. Proteins also determine to what degree its passenger cholesterol and other lipids will interact and be deposited into plaque. In other words, *it is the protein component of the particle that determines the behavior of the lipoprotein particle.* The cholesterol component just goes along for the ride.

When your cholesterol is tested in your doctor's office or hospital, the amount of cholesterol present is measured, while the protein component is ignored. This approach assumes that all cholesterol is the same and ignores the important fact that behavior of a cholesterol particle depends on its protein partner. When you are told that your LDL cholesterol is 150, this means that the amount of cholesterol in the LDL (low-density lipoprotein) fraction is 150 (actually 150 milligrams in 100 milliliters of blood, or 150 mg/dl). The problem is that the low-density lipoproteins are actually composed of a *varied mixture of particle types* that differ in potential for causing heart disease. You simply cannot judge this from knowing that the LDL cholesterol is 150 mg/dl. Likewise, when you're told your HDL is 45 mg/dl, this really means that the cholesterol in the HDL fraction of blood is 45. Like LDL, HDL is also a heterogeneous mixture of particles.

Until recently, measuring lipoproteins was a cumbersome process available only in research laboratories. Testing technology has advanced considerably and several methods are now widely available. The two most commonly used methods used to measure lipoproteins are "electropheresis" and "nuclear magnetic resonance (NMR) spectroscopy".

Drs. Ronald Krauss and Robert Superko of the University of California-San Francisco and Berkeley HeartLabs are among the two leading physician researchers who have explored and popularized the use of electropheresis to study lipoproteins. In this technique, your blood (plasma) is placed in a gel subjected to an electrical charge. Lipoproteins migrate through the gel in patterns that depend on size and electrical charge. The amount of lipoproteins within various classes is then measured. This method has been validated by hundreds of scientific publications.

A newer technique is NMR spectroscopy. Using a device similar to that used to image the body (MRI), a magnetic field is applied to blood (plasma). Physicist Dr. James Otvos of LipoScience, Inc. developed the background science to understand how a magnetic field reveals what kinds and amounts of lipoproteins are present. NMR is quick (performed in minutes), not dependent on the skill of the technician (who simply inserts the blood sample into the device), and is inexpensive (about 50% of the cost of electropheresis). NMR also provides several helpful pieces of information not provided by other methods (such as very low density lipoproteins, or VLDL, and intermediate density lipoproteins, or IDL). Even after using this technology for several years, I am still in awe at the genius of this elegant technique.

Can I "get by" with just lipids?

If you are unable or unwilling to have your lipoproteins tested, what sort of success can you expect relying on lipids alone? This varies, depending on whether you do or don't have multiple causes of plaque not revealed by lipids (such as lipoprotein (a), homocysteine, small LDL, etc., all discussed in the next chapter). It is reasonable, however, to begin with a therapeutic program based on your lipid results. You and your doctor can then tailor your treatment based on the **Track Your Plaque** concept of a repeat heart scan score. In another words, if your score stops increasing or decreases based only on lipid management, you've succeeded. But if your score goes up, particularly 20% or more per year, you should seriously reconsider having lipoproteins performed to design a better treatment program. The goal remains the same: keep your score from increasing.

Some people ask if just lowering LDL cholesterol to very low levels is sufficient to control their plaque. Fueling this argument are clinical trials like the

"PROVE IT" Trial published in early 2004 by Dr. Christopher Cannon of Harvard, in which high dose atorvastatin (Lipitor), 80 mg, was pitted head-to-head against pravastatin (Pravachol), 40 mg, in people recovering from heart attack or unstable heart symptoms (unstable angina). The trial was designed to compare a high intensity LDL lowering strategy against a low intensity therapy. Atorvastatin lowered LDL to 62 mg/dl, while pravastatin lowered LDL to 95 mg/dl. This change resulted in a 16% greater reduction in events with the atorvastatin. However, even at a LDL cholesterol of 62 mg/dl in the subjects taking atorvastatin, 22% of them still experienced death, repeat heart attack, or required major procedures. Intensive LDL lowering may therefore be better, but it is still *not* the final answer.

Likewise, it is not generally sufficient to drop LDL to really low levels and expect that your heart scan score drops, also. Most people do require attention to more than LDL. Only an occasional participant who starts with a very high HDL (>60 mg/dl) and no hidden lipoprotein patterns will enjoy dramatic drops in their score relying only on LDL lowering therapies.

The concept of lipoproteins represents a major advance in understanding the causes behind atherosclerotic coronary disease. As powerful as lipoproteins are, do they tell you whether or not you have coronary plaque present? No, we still rely on Step 1 of **Track Your Plaque,** your heart scan score, to tell us this. Lipids and lipoproteins represent Step 2 of **Track Your Plaque** and provide insight into the causes of heart disease.

In chapter 8, we will discuss the individual lipid and lipoprotein risk factors that can be measured and used as tools for treatment for your **Track Your Plaque** program.

Summary

Too often, relying on cholesterol to identify the risk for future heart attack is no better than a gamble with the odds stacked against you. Most people with heart disease, in fact, have *multiple* causes of coronary plaque which may or may not include high cholesterol. Once hidden coronary plaque is detected and quantified, you will need to identify its causes, so that you are equipped with tools to gain control of plaque growth. Assessment of lipoproteins is the method of choice to pinpoint many of the causes of coronary plaque and thereby lead to more powerful tools for your prevention program.

Track Your Plaque

Step 3

Chapter 8

LDL cholesterol and beyond: The many causes of heart disease and their treatments

How lipoproteins make the causes of coronary plaque seem obvious

Step 2 of **Track Your Plaque** is to pinpoint the causes of your coronary plaque. We accomplish this through lipid and lipoprotein testing. These tests do not tell us whether or not you have plaque, but help identify how plaque started and continues to grow. We will then use treatment of your lipid and/or lipoprotein abnormalities as the hammers and chisels to chip away at your coronary plaque. Because the identification of lipid and lipoprotein disorders is so closely tied to their treatments, this chapter blends both Steps 2 and 3 **Track Your Plaque.**

This chapter serves as a starting place to appreciate the potential abnormalities that can be identified, as well as beginning a discussion about treatment. To get to Step 3, correction of lipid/lipoprotein abnormalities, the involvement of your physician will be required, so I would encourage you to discuss your treatment program with the physician you choose to work with. (See Appendix C for resources to help find a doctor willing to work with you in the event your present physician is unable or unwilling to do so.)

We'll begin with the measures included in the standard lipid panel: LDL cholesterol, HDL cholesterol, and triglycerides. We'll then further explore the concept of lipoprotein testing for those of you interested in a more precise and powerful approach.

LDL cholesterol

Despite its deficiencies in identifying people with heart disease, LDL cholesterol is still a useful tool for treatment. Volumes of clinical data support the concept of LDL lowering to reduce (though not eliminate) heart attack risk.

How low should LDL be if you have an abnormal heart scan score? Most authorities suggest that LDL cholesterol should be lowered to <100 mg/dl if you have a history of heart attack, stent, or bypass surgery. In **Track Your Plaque,** we try even harder. The LDL level that maximizes the likelihood of plaque shrinkage is 60 mg/dl. The majority of our participants who've succeeded in the program, in fact, manage to keep LDL in the 50-60 range. Reducing LDL cholesterol to this level does not guarantee that plaque will not grow, but does make it much more likely.

Dietary strategies that lower LDL cholesterol include avoiding sources of saturated fat, hydrogenated fats, and increasing intake of complex fibers (discussed in greater detail in chapter 9). Raw almonds and walnuts, starchy beans (Spanish, black, kidney, lima, etc.), pectin sources like citrus peels and apples, and psyllium seed (Metamucil)are particularly effective fiber sources that can lower LDL 10%. Oat bran is a versatile fiber source that packs a greater LDL lowering punch than oatmeal when you add three tablespoons per day to yogurt, cottage cheese, protein drinks, etc. or use it as a hot cereal itself. Soy protein powder, generally purchased as one lb. canisters at health food or grocery stores, is a great supplement that you can add to protein shakes, yogurt, oatmeal, etc. Three tablespoons daily can lower LDL around 15%. The butter substitutes Take Control and Benecol contain soybean oil-derived phytosterols that can lower LDL around 10% when you use two tablespoons each day.

The statin class of drugs are very effective in lowering LDL cholesterol with low risk. Though not a requirement to control your heart scan score, the statin agents can surely make life easier getting your LDL to goal if you start with a LDL of >130 mg/dl. Drops in LDL of 30–40% are easily achieved with maximum effects of around 60%. Ezetimibe (Zetia) is an effective non-statin prescription agent that lowers LDL around 18%, or can be used to triple or quadruple the potency of your statin drug.

There are a number of nutritional supplements purported to lower LDL cholesterol that are discussed further in chapter 11. However, our experience with supplements like red yeast, policosanol, pantetheine, and gugulipid has been disappointing. The most effective supplements are listed above, particularly fiber sources and soy protein powder.

HDL cholesterol

HDL is our friend, a protective class of lipoproteins responsible for a process called reverse cholesterol transport, or scavenging cholesterol from plaque. HDL is critically important for regression of plaque.

A low HDL (below 40 mg/dl) is among the most common causes for heart disease. Of every 100 people with heart disease, at least 50 have a low HDL. It is a common cause of heart disease in many people who've been told that either they have no reason for heart disease, or they have a cause that is untreatable. Both statements are simply untrue.

A low HDL is the tip of the iceberg for several other closely-related abnormalities. People who have a low HDL commonly also have a smorgasbord of small LDL particles, high triglycerides, and abnormal triglyceride-rich lipoproteins called VLDL (very low density lipoprotein). HDL is very sensitive to body weight. As you gain weight, HDL plummets. Conversely, weight-loss causes it to increase. A low HDL can also be a marker for the potential for hypertension (high blood pressure), glucose intolerance (pre-diabetes), and full-blown diabetes. (This combination is often called the metabolic syndrome, or syndrome X.) Expression of hypertension and diabetes are also highly weight sensitive.

For **Track Your Plaque,** we aim to raise HDL to 60 mg/dl or greater. This appears to be the *minimum* level necessary to gain control of your score.

How do you raise HDL? Diet can help a great deal. But a standard low-fat diet does not raise HDL, and super low-fat diets *lower* HDL, worsens the small LDL size abnormality, raises triglycerides, and increases VLDL particles—all of which *heighten* your risk of heart disease. People with a low HDL or any of the other associated abnormalities do better with specific modifications in diet that we will discuss in more detail in chapter 9, such as using foods rich in monounsaturated fatty acids (like raw nuts and olive oil), selecting low glycemic index (less sugar-raising) foods, and increasing protein intake.

Exercise raises HDL. Going from a sedentary lifestyle to a moderately active lifestyle (walking 30 minutes per day five days a week) typically raises total HDL two to five points. This effect lasts about two weeks after exercise stops before your HDL drifts back down. Exercise therefore needs to be consistent and long-term in order to prop up your HDL. Most people with low HDL can raise it about 5–10 points with a combination of changes in diet and exercise.

There's a lack of truly effective supplements to raise HDL, and we could really use better tools. Fish oil can have a modest effect in raising HDL, but is more effective in shifting to larger particle size. We frequently, therefore, resort to medical treatments to raise HDL. These treatments are identical to those

that are used to treat the small LDL particle size (see below). The only difference is that raising HDL in some people may require somewhat higher doses of
niacin or other agents.

Triglycerides

Triglycerides are among the four measures included in the standard lipid
panel. Triglycerides can be a very tough customer to figure out. When they're
high, they may or may not cause coronary disease; when they're low, they may
or may not cause coronary disease. Can we make sense out of this jumble?

For the most part, you and I are most interested in triglyceride levels of up to
400 mg/dl, as this is the range that tends to contribute to growth of coronary
plaque. When triglycerides are greater than 400, your doctor will need to consider whether several other conditions might be to blame, such as unknown or
poorly controlled diabetes, an under active thyroid, kidney disease, or certain
genetic disorders (e.g., familial hypertriglyceridemia). Levels this high may or
may not contribute to heart disease risk (which can be decided when your doctor looks at your LDL particle number or apoprotein B, discussed below). In the
rare instances when triglycerides >1000, the pancreas (in your abdomen) can
suffer damage. Levels this high need to be urgently addressed by your doctor.

Triglyceride levels of 100–400 are very common and can contribute significantly to plaque growth. It is also among the most neglected measures in medical practice. What makes triglycerides bad? First of all, triglycerides are present
in virtually all lipoprotein particles to various degrees, such as VLDL and small
LDL. The higher the triglyceride level (up to 400 mg/dl), the greater the quantity of these undesirable lipoprotein particles, all of which are potent causes of
plaque growth. Only when triglycerides are <100 mg/dl can you confidently
predict that triglyceride-containing lipoprotein particles are not present.

Replacing carbohydrate calories (from flour-containing products like
breads, bagels, pasta, and cakes; potatoes; sweets like candy and soft drinks)
with protein and healthy fats like the monounsaturates from raw nuts, olive
and canola oils, or the omega-3s from fish and flaxseed products, will all help
reduce triglycerides. Avoiding processed foods containing high fructose corn
syrup is crucial, as this ubiquitous additive (in everything from low-fat salad
dressings to breads) raises triglycerides significantly. Fish oil supplements (but
not flaxseed oil) can dramatically lower triglycerides. (See chapter 10.) For
Track Your Plaque, everyone is advised to take at least 4000 mg per day of a fish
oil supplement (30% DHA/EPA), with our target triglyceride level being <100
mg/dl. Prescription agents that lower triglycerides include niacin (doses >500

mg, which should be monitored by your physician), the fibrates like gemfi-brozil (Lopid) and fenofibrate (Tricor); and the statin agents, especially ator-vastatin (Lipitor) and rosuvastatin (Crestor).

Total cholesterol

Total cholesterol is mentioned only for completeness. It is a measure that we do *not* use in **Track Your Plaque,** as it is a combination of three measures:

$$\text{Total cholesterol} = \text{LDL} + \text{HDL} + \text{triglycerides} \div 5$$

In other words, if LDL or triglycerides go up, your cholesterol goes up. If HDL goes up (a positive change), cholesterol again *goes up.* Total cholesterol is a composite of these other measures and is therefore too sloppy a measure for us to use. Its only usefulness is in crude screening situations (e.g., at the mall) to identify people with high cholesterol (though the frightfully common low HDL pattern will be completely missed).

Let's move on and discuss the various lipoprotein measures.

LDL particle number, apoprotein B

Remember our discussion of how your doctor measures cholesterol? He/she essentially lets the oil (cholesterol) separate and measures how much there is. This flawed approach neglects the fact that cholesterol really occurs as a pas-senger on lipoprotein particles, i.e, it is only a passive component of a larger blood particle.

One way to improve on this crude practice is to actually *count* the number of lipoprotein particles present in a given volume, say, per cc of blood.

Think of it this way: the more particles there are in your blood, the more likely they will enter the wall of the artery and contribute to plaque forma-tion. Some call this a gradient-driven process. You might recall from high school science class that when a concentration gradient is present across a semi-permeable membrane, it will work towards achieving equilibrium to eliminate the concentration difference. The same principle applies when a higher concentration of LDL particles is present in blood compared to the artery wall (with the thin inner lining of the artery acting as the membrane). The more numerous LDL particles in the blood infiltrate the artery wall in an effort to balance the concentration gradient.

Low LDL cholesterol and high LDL particle number

A very common situation is to have low or "normal" LDL cholesterol but a high LDL particle number or apoprotein B. This situation can lead to plaque growth even though LDL cholesterol is not high.

Tim provides a good example. Tim is a 34-year-old mathematician. Although his parents (in their 60's) didn't have heart problems, his maternal uncles both had heart attacks in their 50s. Tim underwent a heart scan. His score: 30-a low absolute score, but very high for his young age (75-95th percentile). A future of heart disease was inevitable unless we took action.

Tim's lipoprotein profile (NMR) showed:

LDL particle number	2254 nm/l
LDL cholesterol	124 mg/dl
HDL cholesterol	31 mg/dl
Triglycerides	360 mg/dl

(Tim also showed severe abnormalities of VLDL particles; intermediate density lipoproteins, and a complete shift of LDL particles to the undesirable small fraction.)

One of the principal causes of Tim's coronary plaque was his high LDL particle number (in the worst 10% of people) *even though his LDL cholesterol was favorable* (below the average range).

LDL particle number is one of the most powerful tools we have available. It can be measured directly as LDL particle number (by the NMR method) or apoprotein B, which is more widely available. (We will use LDL particle number and apoprotein B interchangeably in our discussion.) The Quebec Cardiovascular Study, a large Canadian study conducted in the 1990's, is the most convincing demonstration of how apoprotein B was the best lipid/lipoprotein predictor of heart attack. In this study and several others like it, heart attack still occurred even when LDL cholesterol was low but apoprotein B was high. In other words, apoprotein B proved a superior indicator of heart attack potential, even when LDL cholesterol was low. (See box.)

You cannot predict LDL particle number or apoprotein B by just looking at LDL cholesterol. In other words, you can have a high LDL particle number with low LDL cholesterol, a low LDL particle number with low LDL cholesterol, etc. LDL particle number or apoprotein B needs to be specifically measured.

How can LDL cholesterol be low when particle number is high? The amount of cholesterol contained per particle varies widely. If your LDL particles have less cholesterol in each particle but there are many of them, the measured LDL cholesterol may remain low, but your heart disease risk will be high (because of the high particle number and the resultant concentration gradient.)

There are many people with established heart disease who've been told their LDL cholesterol was fine, and that no cause for their heart disease could be identified. Many people like this have excessively high LDL particle numbers or apoprotein B (often, though not always, combined with a low HDL).

You can still have a heart attack while being treated for a high LDL cholesterol with a statin agent (Zocor, Lipitor, Pravachol, Lescol, Mevacor, Crestor) if your LDL particle number is high. In other words, despite the appearance of a good response to a cholesterol-lowering agent, heart attack can still occur because the number of LDL particles is still excessive.

If you rely only on LDL cholesterol and neglect to measure particle number or apoprotein B, you will be groping in the dark—you won't know if treatment is required nor will you know if treatment is sufficient. You simply need to measure LDL particle number or apoprotein B to know. Reducing saturated and hydrogenated fats in your diet, cholesterol lowering

---

Jack and Walter-Same LDL cholesterols, very different fates

Jack has a LDL cholesterol of 124 mg/dl. "Not bad!" his doctor says. His friend Walter also has a LDL of 124. Jack has a major heart attack at age 53. Walter never has a heart attack.

How can two men with identical LDL's have such different fates?

Walter's lipoprotein analysis showed a normal LDL particle size and a low number of LDL particles (low apoprotein B). Jack's analysis, on the other hand, showed abnormally small LDL particles and a high number of LDL particles—*small particles and too many of them.*

Despite the very same LDL cholesterols, these two men have extremely different risks for heart disease, with Jack's very high risk conferred by a high number of small LDL particles.

---

drugs, and several dietary strategies all reduce LDL particle number and apoprotein B. These are the same treatments that lower LDL cholesterol. (See above.) For participants in **Track Your Plaque,** our targets for treatment that enhance likelihood of stopping plaque growth are an LDL particle number of <700 or an apoprotein B of 60 mg/dl or less.

Small LDL particle size

Just like people, LDL particles come in a variety of sizes—some big, some small, some in-between. Children are more likely to have healthy, large LDL particles. Small particles become more common as we age. Small LDL particles can double or triple the likelihood of developing coronary plaque and heart attack. Small LDL is an inherited trait unmasked by unhealthy lifestyles and excessive body weight, and suppressed by a healthy lifestyle. When the genetic trait is strong, it can even occur in slender, active people with healthy lifestyles. It is among the most common reasons for heart disease, being found in 50% of all people who eventually develop heart attack. It often occurs alongside a low

HDL, though not always. Some call small LDL "LDL pattern B", as distin-guished from "LDL pattern A" with large LDL's.

Like LDL particle number, you can't judge LDL size by just looking at LDL cholesterol. In other words, even if LDL cholesterol is low, particle size can be small (and LDL particle number increased), yet it can still be responsible for building coronary plaque. Small LDL begins to appear when triglycerides are >70 mg/dl or HDL <60 mg/dl. But even HDL and triglycerides often do not tell you with absolute confidence whether or not small LDL is present. It is not uncommon, for instance, to have triglycerides of >400, yet have no small LDL. Conversely, you might have a triglyceride level that's <150 mg/dl, but small LDL can still be present. Like LDL particle number or apoprotein B, LDL size needs to be directly measured.

Small LDL particles are a powerful cause for plaque growth. Smaller particles more readily penetrate artery walls and deposit material into plaques. Small LDL's are also more adherent to structural materials that reside in plaque. They also hang around in the blood longer than larger particles, providing more opportunity to do damage

While small LDL is a bad thing to have, it is usually easy to treat. Weight-loss is a powerful method of increasing LDL size. The amount of weight-loss required to correct LDL size varies widely. Some people can convert back to a large LDL size just by losing 10 pounds. Others may require more, depending on your starting weight and genetics. Exercise also has a modest, though transient effect.

Can you be at your ideal weight, be vigorously active, and still have small LDL particles? Yes, unfortunately, you can. In other words, small LDL is a *genetic* characteristic that is worsened by excess weight and inactivity. But the pattern can be present even when everything appears perfect.

That's when we turn to medical treatments. Niacin (vitamin B3), when used at prescription doses is a very powerful way to correct LDL size. Doses of 1000–2000 mg are very effective, depending on your weight and some genetic factors. Niacin is best prescribed by a doctor who has experience in dealing with the peculiar effects of niacin (most of them harmless), like feeling hot and itchy. Unfortunately, many patients and physicians are unnecessarily scared by these effects and give up. If weight-loss and exercise have failed to achieve full correction of the small LDL pattern, niacin is first choice. (Prescription long-acting "Niaspan", made by Kos Pharmaceuticals is preferred. This preparation is less likely to provoke the typical "hot-flash" sensation characteristic of niacin.) Niacin is the most likely to completely eliminate small LDL.

Please be advised that niacin is best taken under medical supervision. You can try to take niacin over-the-counter, but people who try this route rarely manage to achieve the doses required to fully correct their abnormalities because of intolerable flushing. Liver side-effects are rare with the Niaspan preparation, but it is wise to have your liver tested periodically by your doctor when you're taking any form of niacin (usually every six months). Avoid over-the-counter slow-release niacin preparations, as these preparations do carry significant risk of liver toxicity, unlike the prescription formulation.

Other agents for your doctor to consider are the fibric acid derivatives (also prescription medicines—Lopid (gemfibrozil) and Tricor (fenofibrate); the glitazones—Actos (rosiglitazone) and Avandia (pioglitazone); and Pletal (cilostazol), ordinarily used for claudication, or poor circulation to the legs. These are non-FDA approved applications and need to be thoroughly discussed with your doctor. The statin cholesterol medicines have no significant specific effect on small LDL.

As with low HDL, there is a lack of helpful nutritional tools that increase LDL size. Omega-3 fatty acids in fish oil do increase LDL size, but only to a very modest degree. (See chapter 10.) The only food beyond fish oil that increases LDL particle size is oat bran. Oat bran is a great adjunctive strategy that lowers LDL cholesterol and particle number, and also increases LDL particle size. (Also discussed further in chapter 10.) Oat bran is inexpensive, versatile, and available just about anywhere. Use oat bran by adding 2-3 tablespoons a day to yogurt, fruit smoothies, cereal, or to your cooking.

Should you have small LDL particles identified as one of the causes of your heart disease, set yourself on a course of action: increase physical activity, lose weight when appropriate, add supplements like fish oil and oat bran, and consider treatments that increase the particle size and turn-off this potent abnormality. All these efforts will also increase HDL. Just as you often cannot tell whether you have small LDL particles at the start of your program, you will likewise not be able to gauge whether it's been eliminated until you measure it again. Another test of LDL particle size will eventually be necessary to assess treatment effects.

HDL subclasses

Like LDL, HDL is really a collection of different particles. We call the entire family "total HDL". The truly effective HDL that participates in reverse cholesterol transport that may shrink plaque is large HDL, sometimes also known as HDL2b. In other words, not all HDL is beneficial; only the large HDL particles are truly helpful. The smaller fractions can comprise a major portion of total HDL, and a seemingly favorable HDL of, say, 50 can conceal a serious lack of effective large HDL's.

Unlike LDL, you can make some preliminary judgments about HDL size based on total HDL. Above a total HDL of 60 mg/dl, large HDL is confidently in a good range. Below 40 mg/dl, and you can be very confident that there is a deficiency of large HDL. Between a total HDL of 40 and 60 is an indeterminate range, and you may or may not have a lack of large HDL. This is where measuring HDL size is most helpful.

In **Track Your Plaque**, we try to keep your large HDL at least 50% of the total (by NMR) or 30% HDL2b (by electropheresis), aiming for a total HDL of 60 mg/dl or greater. You can increase the proportion of large HDL by using the same treatment strategies as those used to correct the small LDL abnormality (above). A lack of large HDL is a relatively easy abnormality to treat, but you just have to recognize whether it's present and whether it is fully corrected with your treatment efforts.

Very low-density lipoprotein (VLDL)

VLDL particles are lipoproteins produced by the liver, larger and richer in triglycerides than LDL particles. VLDL loves to share its plentiful triglycerides with other particles. This is the process that leads to the formation of small LDL and small HDL particles. Although VLDL are essentially triglyceride carrying lipoproteins, you can have an excessive quantity of large VLDL even with low triglycerides.

The dangers of triglyceride containing particles are therefore not fully evident from the triglyceride level on a lipid panel. Though you're probably safe if triglycerides are <100 mg/dl, enough VLDL can occasionally be present even at this level to contribute triglycerides to other particles and produce the small LDL and HDL patterns.

The treatment of excessive VLDL is the same as for triglycerides (above). Fish oil is an especially helpful way to lower VLDL, with significant reductions beginning at 4000 mg/day (of a 30% EPA/DHA preparation). As with the question of LDL and LDL particle number, knowing your VLDL gives you a better handle on which treatments to consider and whether your treatment is sufficient, even when triglycerides appear favorable.

Intermediate-density lipoprotein (IDL)

You've heard of *low* density lipoproteins (LDL) and *high* density lipoproteins (HDL). Let me introduce you to *intermediate* density lipoproteins, or IDL. IDL is a very potent cause of heart disease. It is usually lumped together with LDL in conventional lipid panels and not individually measured, so you won't know you have it if you relied just on these numbers. A high IDL means that your body struggles to clear fat from the blood after you eat, with many more hours required to clear the blood than normal. The longer these particles persist in the blood, the more opportunity they have to interact with the artery wall and cause plaque growth.

IDL is available through an NMR panel. (It is not available with the electropheretic panel.) Only about 10% of people with heart disease have an elevated IDL. This abnormality responds to a broad variety of treatments, including cholesterol lowering medicines, niacin, fish oil, and weight-loss. Knowing that you have a high IDL may mean your treatment needs to be intensified, as IDL may persist even when LDL or other parameters appear corrected. The **Track Your Plaque** goal is zero milligrams of IDL in your fasting blood.

> **Track Your Plaque approach to treatment of Lp (a):**
> 1) Lower LDL cholesterol to 60 mg/dl or lower.
> 2) Lower LDL particle number to <700 (nm/l) or apoprotein B <60 mg/dl.
> 3) Normalize LDL particle size, i.e., eliminate the small LDL particle tendency.
> 4) Raise HDL to >60 mg/dl and normalize the HDL subtype distribution.
> 5) Lower Lp (a) to less than 30 mg/dl (which in most laboratories represents the upper limit of normal; this may require modification, depending on the lab you select.), choosing from niacin, l-carnitine, CoQ10, raw almonds, flaxseed, and fish oil.
> 6) Correct endothelial dysfunction, usually accomplished with supplemental l-arginine or medication (such as ACE inhibitors, a class of medicines for high blood pressure).
> 7) Aggressive correction of hypertension, including normalizing a hypertensive response to exercise.
> 8) Consider addition of estrogen (peri- or post-menopausal females) or testosterone (males).
>
> This approach is only a suggested strategy. However, our experience in using your heart scan score as a measure of success or failure suggests that this broad, albeit complicated, approach is the most effective to keep plaque from growing when Lp(a) is part of the picture.

Lipoprotein (a)

Lipoprotein (a), or Lp (a) (read "L-P little a"), is a very powerful cause of premature heart disease. Lp (a) is often responsible for heart attacks in young people, commonly women in their 50s and men in their 40s. About 17% of people with heart disease have increased Lp (a). It is also one of the greatest challenges to treat and perhaps the one we struggle with the most, along with the metabolic syndrome.

Lp (a) is actually an LDL particle with an additional protein attached, called apoprotein a. Lp (a) magnifies the dangers of all other abnormalities, especially LDL. Lp(a) is unusual in that it has a dual dangerous effect. It encourages plaque growth, as well as blood clot formation when plaque ruptures. Lp (a) is also a potent cause of endothelial dysfunction, a fancy name for abnormal constriction of arteries. When Lp(a) causes endothelial dysfunction, arterial injury results that contributes to further plaque growth. High blood pressure is very common with Lp (a) and is probably related to abnormal constriction of arteries throughout the body. People who have Lp(a) commonly have significant high blood pressure in their late 50s or 60s. This, in turn, causes even more damage to the artery wall and encourages plaque growth.

Lp (a) is a genetic trait that you inherit from either your mom or dad, and you pass on to each of your children with 50:50 likelihood. For this reason, if you have Lp (a), you should consider advising your grown children to be tested, particularly if they are over 30 years old.

Treatment for Lp (a) is controversial. Most experts agree that, at the very least, LDL cholesterol should be aggressively lowered to a level no higher than 80 mg/dl., usually using a statin drug, thought Lp(a) itself will not be lowered by this effort. Specific suppression of Lp(a) is most effectively accomplished with niacin, though in higher doses than that used to correct small LDL or increase HDL. Higher doses should only be taken under supervision of a physician because of the greater likelihood of side-effects. In females, estrogen preparations may lower Lp(a), generally around 25%. Of course, estrogen use has been recognized as having both positive and negative effects. In the HERS trial of post-menopausal estrogen use, while there was no overall benefit to most women, the only exception was in participants with Lp(a), who did benefit by lowering heart attack risk. This is an important conversation to have with your family doctor or gynecologist. For men, testosterone can lower Lp(a) approximately 25%. (Both estrogen preparations and testosterone are prescription drugs.)

There are several nutritional supplements and foods that lower Lp(a) including raw almonds, flaxseed, coenzyme Q10, and fish oil, though the magnitude of Lp(a) reduction is modest; these are all discussed in further detail in chapter 11. Given the difficulty in lowering Lp(a), it's worth considering several of these supplements if you have this abnormality. L-carnitine is an amino acid that is also useful for lowering Lp(a). A dose of 2000 mg per day (usually as 1000 mg twice a day) lowers Lp(a) 15–20% and is safe and easily tolerated.

The **Track Your Plaque** approach to Lp (a), though more complex than treatments for other lipoprotein disorders (see box), proceeds with the same goal as for other abnormalities. We first begin a treatment program, then adjust treatment to arrest the growth of plaque, i.e., until your heart scan score no longer increases, or a reduction in score is achieved. In this way, you and your doctor can add or subtract agents or intensify your program, depending on whether you've gained control of your plaque.

Homocysteine

For years, Dr. Kilmer McCully of Harvard Medical School argued that homocysteine represents a major risk factor for heart disease. The whole idea began when it was observed that children with a rare metabolic disorder called homocystinuria developed aggressive coronary disease in their teens and twenties. These unfortunate young people had very high levels of homocysteine in the blood (often >200 mmol/l), as well as high levels in their urine (thus the name "homocystinuria"). Further study, including extensive work by Dr. McCully, led to the finding that coronary disease could be related to lesser levels of homocysteine. People appeared to develop heart disease as adults with homocysteine levels in the 20–50 range. Several large epidemiologic studies have confirmed that homocysteine levels even above 10 are associated with a three-fold increase in heart attack risk. Homocysteine injures artery walls, oxidizes LDL particles (making them more damaging), causes endothelial dysfunction (abnormal constriction of arteries), and encourages blood clot formation, leading to heart attack. Approximately 10–20% of all people with heart disease will have homocysteine levels >10.

Most of the data that support the idea of homocysteine as a cause of coronary plaque accumulation is epidemiologic, i.e, based on observing large numbers of people with varying levels of homocysteine to see whether it predicts heart attack. There is a lack of research on the effects of treatment, however. The closest we have to a persuasive argument for the benefits of treatment is two trials following coronary angioplasty, with a marked reduction in heart attack and similar events when people with higher homocysteine levels were treated. Nonetheless, the existing epidemiologic observations are so compelling and the treatment safe and simple that correcting elevated homocysteine levels is easily justified.

Treatment of a high homocysteine (>10) consists of vitamins B6 (25–100 mg), B12 (500 mcg or more), and folic acid (1–5 mg), all B vitamins. Folic acid can be obtained in doses up to 0.8 mg (800 micrograms) over-the-counter. Higher doses of 1.0 mg or greater are available only by prescription but generally necessary only when homocysteine levels exceed 18 mmol/l. Be careful not to use more than 100 mg of vitamin B6, as this is one of the vitamins that, when used in too high a dose, can cause peripheral neuropathy (nervous system dysfunction). Your doctor will also need to think about vitamin B12 deficiency, particularly if folic acid alone is used. Very rarely, administration of folic acid unmasks hidden vitamin B12 deficiency, causing a red tongue, a specific sort of anemia, and neurologic effects.

C-reactive protein

C-reactive protein (CRP) is just one of a family of markers that we can use to measure the body's inflammatory state. If inflammatory white blood cells are active in some part of the body—joints, lung, colon, etc., as well as plaque in coronary arteries—C-reactive protein (produced by the liver) will be increased. Inflammation increases the likelihood that plaque ruptures its surface covering, exposing the underlying contents and provoking blood clot formation and heart attack. An elevated CRP suggests that inflammation may be ongoing in your coronary plaque.

You can immediately see a difficulty here. If there is inflammation *anywhere* in the body, CRP levels will be increased. For this reason, measures of inflammation are best applied in the well, asymptomatic person who does not have some obvious source of inflammation like arthritis or colitis, recent surgery, recent infection, etc. In these people, very high CRP's are meaningless from a heart standpoint. In apparently well people, however, modest elevations of CRP can suggest hidden inflammation in the plaque of your coronary arteries. For this reason, a newer method of measuring CRP, called high sensitivity CRP, has been developed that can detect subtle elevations that can signify increased coronary plaque inflammation. While levels >10 nearly always represent inflammation outside of the heart and should not be used to prognosticate coronary risk, lower levels (usually <4) can be used to gauge coronary plaque inflammation.

Dr. Paul Ridker of Harvard University is a noted authority on CRP. He has convincingly shown that high CRP levels, and therefore greater levels of plaque inflammation, pose up to three-fold higher risk of heart attack, even when LDL cholesterol is low. When both CRP and LDL cholesterol are high, then risk is even greater. When an elevated CRP occurs in the company of small LDL particle size, an especially high risk for heart attack is present, increased as much as six to seven-fold.

An interesting study from UCLA explored heart attack risk posed by the combination of CRP and coronary calcium score. Participants in this study who had both low CRP's and low EBT scores (<4) had a very low risk for heart attack and death. Participants at the opposite extreme with a high CRP (highest quarter) and high calcium scores (>142) had 7.5-fold greater risk. Interestingly, participants with low calcium scores (<4) but high CRP's had only a minimal increase in heart attack risk. This makes sense: How can you rupture plaque if you have little or no plaque to inflame and rupture?

The treatment of a high CRP is still being sorted out. Most research suggests that statin agents used to lower LDL cholesterol lower CRP within a few months of starting treatment. The recently approved agent ezetimibe (Zetia) also lowers CRP by about 10–20%. Aspirin and fish oil, because they have anti-inflammatory properties, also lower CRP. A diet rich in fiber, particularly oat products, raw almonds, and psyllium seed (Metamucil), can have a significant CRP lowering effect. Weight-loss and exercise also reduce CRP.

In a practical sense, if you have an elevated CRP, you should be regarded as being at higher risk for heart attack, even in the absence of other lipid or lipoprotein abnormalities. Efforts to reduce CRP might be considered, such as a statin agent, fish oil, dietary fiber, weight-loss and exercise. The only time you might *not* have to take an elevated CRP level seriously is if your EBT score is 0 or very low (<10).

Fibrinogen

Fibrinogen is a blood protein that, when present in excessive levels, can lead to blood clotting. As you now know, when an atherosclerotic plaque in a coronary artery ruptures, plaque contents are exposed to flowing blood. Interestingly, not every plaque that ruptures results in heart attack. If the tendency to form a blood clot is not sufficiently powerful, the ruptured plaque may heal, no blood clot forms and therefore no blockage of blood flow results. This can all happen without your awareness. However, if excessive fibrinogen or other clotting proteins are present, a blood clot forms and plugs the artery closed within minutes, resulting in heart attack.

Poor diet and physical inactivity raise fibrinogen blood levels to unhealthy levels. Estrogen also raises fibrinogen levels, which may account for some of the increased blood clotting tendency observed with estrogen replacement in post-menopausal women (such as blood clots in the leg and pelvic veins, as well as heart attack).

Fibrinogen can also promote plaque growth without rupture, but how this occurs is not clear. Fibrinogen is another risk factor that, like Lp(a), can magnify the dangers of other abnormalities. For instance, in the ECAT Study (The European Concerted Action on Thrombosis and Disabilities Angina Pectoris Study, 1995), people who had a combined elevation of LDL cholesterol with a high fibrinogen had a five-fold higher risk of heart attack.

Fibrinogen levels should not exceed 350 mg/dl. There is no specific fibrinogen lowering medicine or supplement (and perhaps this is why we hear so little about it). Fish oil, however, does a pretty good job of lowering fibrinogen and is the preferred treatment. Doses of 4000 mg or greater per day (30% EPA/DHA) are required. Combine this with a diet rich in green vegetables and low in saturated and hydrogenated fat, all of which also lower fibrinogen, and levels usually drop into favorable range. For the occasional person who requires more intensive effort, the fibric acid class of drugs (especially fenofibrate) can lower fibrinogen 15–40%. Niacin can also lower fibrinogen 10–30%.

The role of measuring and treating other clotting proteins is still unclear and we await data on such measures as von Willebrand factor, factor VII, plasminogen activator inhibitor-1, and others.

Goodbye lipid panel?

If lipoproteins are so superior, do we even need to bother with plain old lipids (LDL cholesterol, HDL cholesterol, triglycerides, and total cholesterol)?

If your lipoprotein abnormality is _____.	You can use _____ to assess treatment
Small LDL	HDL , triglycerides
Low large HDL	HDL (total)
VLDL	HDL, triglycerides
LDL particle number, apoprotein B	LDL cholesterol

In Step 2 of **Track Your Plaque**, a full lipoprotein analysis is the preferred method to *diagnose* how your coronary plaque was caused. Lipoprotein analysis is also the best way to determine whether, after treatments have been introduced, the abnormalities have been fully corrected. Simple lipids (not lipoproteins) are still useful *to monitor the effects of treatment* along the way, even if your abnormalities were not fully evident on initial lipid testing.

Let me explain. While Steps 1 and 2 of **Track Your Plaque** can be completed in a matter of days, Step 3, or correction of your lipoprotein disorders, often requires several months and adjustments of the dose or type of treatment. The easiest and least expensive way to monitor response to treatment is to perform simple lipid measures. In other words, lipids can serve as milestones along the way before you reach your final destination of full correction of lipoprotein abnormalities.

For instance, a common situation is a person with a low total HDL (<40 mg/dl), high triglycerides (>200 mg/dl), increased VLDL, and an abundance of small LDL particles. This person is advised to make diet changes, lose 10 pounds through a carbohydrate restriction, take 4000 mg of fish oil, and begin niacin treatment. After two months, a lipid panel is checked to assess whether there has been the expected change in HDL or triglycerides. Lipid panels are readily available in just about any clinic or hospital laboratory. In this example, if the lipid panel shows an increase in HDL cholesterol and a drop in triglycerides, then the quantity of small LDL particles has also decreased, as these three parameters all respond together and to a similar degree. Perhaps the HDL has increased to 48 and the triglycerides are 187. Both are better, but not yet to our goals of an HDL of 60 and triglycerides <100, and so the niacin dose is increased by 500 mg, perhaps adding another 2000 mg of fish oil, then another lipid profile is scheduled in a month to again assess the results. In this way, we can use the readily available and inexpensive lipid panels to obtain feedback on whether the desired effects are being achieved.

Similarly, LDL particle number and apoprotein B respond the same as LDL cholesterol. In this way, we can easily and readily gauge whether treatment is yielding the effects we desire, just by doing a simple lipid panel. Other such patterns that can be used to gauge the effects of treatment are shown in the box.

In **Track Your Plaque,** we aim for a LDL cholesterol of 60 mg/dl or less, an HDL of 60 mg/dl or greater, and a triglyceride level of 100 mg/dl or less. Once lipids are where you and your doctor would like them, then the full lipoprotein panel can be checked again. This approach simplifies the work required, since full lipoprotein analysis is required only in the beginning and to assess whether you've achieved your lipoprotein goals. It also cuts down on the need for the somewhat more expensive lipoprotein testing.

Lipoproteins—How to get them in your neighborhood

If you've decided to pursue the lipoprotein route, you will need to work with a physician who has invested the time and effort to be educated on these methods and knows how to use them in clinical practice. Thankfully, more and more physicians are recognizing the deficiencies of conventional lipids and have turned to lipoprotein testing for better answers. You will, therefore, need to locate a physician near you to help obtain testing and provide interpretation. This physician should also offer recommendations regarding potential therapies for your lipoprotein abnormalities. He/she may also help monitor treatment with periodic lipid tests and decide when a lipoprotein re-evaluation is in order.

A listing of resources to help you obtain these tests in your area will be found in Appendix C. If you would like to help your own doctor become better informed on lipoprotein testing, you might begin by referring him/her to these resources. Both testing companies support professional education and recognize that an understanding of lipoproteins does not occur overnight. They will also help your doctor educate his/her staff or the laboratory's staff on how to prepare your blood specimen before submitting it for lipoprotein testing.

Lipoprotein testing is fairly well covered by health insurance. The initial panel that we obtain on **Track Your Plaque** patients (using NMR spectroscopy, LipoScience) costs a total of around $300 (around $90 for basic NMR; $210 for the additional tests). The Berkeley HeartLab service is approximately twice that. Some insurers may not be familiar with lipoprotein testing and occasionally require justification from the ordering physician. Most insurance companies will cover most or all of the cost when appropriate rationale is provided. Even if you are among the few whose insurance will not cover the cost, you can usually persuade them to contribute at least the cost of a conventional lipid panel (ranging from $10 to $100) towards the lipoprotein costs.

Can I rely on plain old lipids?

If you simply are unable or unwilling to get lipoprotein testing, what sort of success can you have relying on simple lipids alone? This varies, depending on whether or not there are multiple hidden causes for your coronary plaque. If you choose to begin with the lipid route, it is reasonable to correct the lipid abnormalities, then repeat your heart scan score (approximately a year later) and assess the results. If your score is unchanged or lower, you've succeeded using lipids alone. But if the rate of increase in score is >20%, you may have hidden abnormalities that should be uncovered by lipoprotein testing. A more intensive effort to obtain these tests will more than likely be rewarded with greater success in achieving control of your plaque.

Track Your Plaque suggested lipoprotein panels

This is a list of the components of the basic lipoprotein panel we've used successfully for tracking and controlling plaque. If you and your doctor choose to use NMR (LipoScience, Inc.), the panel should include:

- LDL particle number
- LDL, HDL, triglycerides, total cholesterol
- LDL, HDL, VLDL, and IDL particle size profiles
- Lipoprotein (a)
- Homocysteine
- C-reactive protein (high-sensitivity assay)

If you go through Berkeley HeartLabs, Inc.("gradient gel electropheresis"), the panel should include:

- LDL gradient gel electrophoresis (LDL GGE)
- HDL gradient gel electrophoresis (HDL GGE)
- LDL, HDL, triglycerides, total cholesterol
- Apoprotein B
- Lipoprotein (a)
- Homocysteine
- C-reactive protein (high-sensitivity assay)
- Fibrinogen

Fibrinogen is not presently available from the LipoScience laboratory but is readily available from most local laboratories. Some additional measures that assess the presence of a borderline diabetic tendency or glucose intolerance can be obtained via NMR or Berkeley or can be obtained locally. (These measures include Hba1C, fasting insulin levels, C-peptide, and fasting glucose. You might consider discussing these measures with your doctor if you have been diagnosed with borderline diabetes, metabolic syndrome, or have been told you have a high blood sugar level.)

How far do we go?

To what degree do lipoproteins need to be corrected?

This can vary depending on your specific pattern of lipoproteins. Ideally, this is best determined by your physician, who can use your heart scan score as the feedback tool to decide whether your lipoproteins have been treated adequately. If your score continues to increase 20% per year or more, then your lipoprotein endpoints definitely require intensification. An increase of 10–20% suggests that modest improvement in your program may be beneficial, e.g., an additional 10% reduction in LDL particle number or apoprotein B, or LDL cholesterol, or a 10% further increase in HDL. If your score has stopped increasing (0% annual change) or, even better, has decreased, then you know that your lipoproteins have been adequately corrected.

To give you and your doctor some reference points for thinking about how to treat your lipoproteins, here is a summary of the endpoints that we've used successfully in **Track Your Plaque:**

Parameter	Treatment Goal
LDL cholesterol	50–60 mg/dl
LDL particle number	<700 nm/l
Small LDL	
NMR	<10 mg/dl
Electropheresis	<15% of total LDL
Apoprotein B	<60 mg/dl
HDL cholesterol	>60 mg/dl
Large HDL	
NMR	>30 mg/dl
Electropheresis	>30% HDL 2b fraction
Triglycerides	<100 mg/dl
VLDL (large)	<7 mg/dl
IDL 0 mg/dl	
Homocysteine	<10 mmol/l
Lipoprotein (a)	<30 mg/dl
C-reactive protein	?

(The endpoints for therapy for C-reactive protein are not well worked out, and so no target value is specified. We await better information.)

Once again, these are only suggested targets. If your heart scan score continues to increase despite achieving these endpoints, you and your doctor should consider treating beyond these suggested goals.

Treatment of your lipid/lipoprotein disorders is Step 3 of your **Track Your Plaque** program. Treatment is specific for each lipoprotein pattern, and so your treatment program needs to be individualized. In chapter 9, we discuss how nutritional strategies can become part of Step 3 of **Track Your Plaque** and can be used to advantage in correcting your lipid/lipoprotein abnormalities, and achieving control of your plaque.

Summary

Step 2 of **Track Your Plaque** is to identify all causes of your coronary plaque. Lipoprotein testing is the most accurate and comprehensive method available to reveal the full extent of abnormalities creating plaque in your coronary arteries. Alternatively, conventional lipids can be used, but should then be treated intensively.

Lipoprotein testing is also the most reliable method for your doctor to determine whether the proper goals have been achieved—lowering LDL particle number sufficiently, lowering homocysteine, etc. To simplify the process along the way, however, readily obtainable lipid panels of LDL, HDL, triglycerides, and total cholesterol, available just about anywhere, can easily and cheaply guide you and your doctor.

Chapter 9

The six Track Your Plaque nutrition principles

Eat right to gain control of your plaque.

People have experimented with just about every kind of diet imaginable: low-fat, ultra-low-fat, high-fat, low-carbohydrate, high-carbohydrate, high-protein, low-protein, vegetarian, Mediterranean, Oriental, rice, grapefruit, Atkin's, Zone, and on and on…

Is there one diet that's right and all the rest are wrong?

Probably not. In fact, every diet fad has taught us something new. The American obsession with diet has amounted to a nationwide experiment in the value (or danger) of various nutritional manipulations. All of these diets have pluses and minuses, strengths and weaknesses. Some lower LDL cholesterol but raise triglycerides, or are unhealthy for other reasons like increasing cancer risk and promoting osteoporosis. Other diets are too restrictive and therefore impractical. Impose too many rules and formulas and people become exasperated, lose interest and drift back to old habits.

To add to the confusion, because people differ genetically, they respond to the same diet differently. A diet that drops one person's LDL cholesterol 30 points and weight 10 lbs. could cause someone else to raise LDL and gain weight.

The diet advocated by the American Heart Association is a modest fat restricted program designed to lower LDL cholesterol by 10%. Surely, we can do better than that. How about an ultra-low-fat diet? In years past, I prescribed the Ornish diet. This program allows <10% of calories from fat sources, compared to 40–45% in the average American diet. People following this diet showed two varying responses: some did well, reducing LDL cholesterol, losing weight, and apparently slowing their heart disease; others enjoyed little or none of these benefits. This larger second group lost little weight, often gained a few pounds, dropped HDL cholesterol and increased triglycerides, and sometimes increased blood sugar into a near diabetic range. When lipoproteins were examined, there was increased small LDL and VLDL. These are changes that encourage *growth* in coronary plaque. In low-fat diets, one size does not fit all.

Can we construct a diet that benefits from these lessons? Is it possible to obtain the benefits we desire yet maintain flexibility and not force you to adhere to strict menus and formulas? Can we use diet effectively in light of lipoprotein analysis and its impact on coronary plaque?

We continue Step 3 of **Track Your Plaque** by discussing the nutrition principles that help correct the causes of plaque as identified by lipid or lipoprotein testing. In subsequent chapters, we will go on to discuss how to use exercise and nutritional supplements.

Not another diet!

The **Track Your Plaque** nutrition program is an eclectic mix of strategies borrowed from many of its predecessors. But don't panic! It is *not* a precisely structured program with percent calories from fat, carbohydrate, etc dictated to you. Instead, it *educates* you about important principles that create *diet habits* that help you succeed in reducing heart disease risk. This approach is flexible, permitting modification to suit personal tastes and heterogeneous lipid/lipoprotein patterns.

10%, 20%, or 30% fat?

First of all, most people simply do not think of food in terms of percent fat, nor can they adhere to formulas dictating what percent of this or that to eat. We might think in terms of fat grams (which we *will* count, at least in the beginning), but most of us in our busy lives just don't bother converting fat intake into percent of total calories. Secondly, precise control over percent fat is probably not that important, but the *type* of fat you eat is crucial. Thirdly, *low-fat* diets often become *high-carbohydrate* diets with an unwanted cascade of lower HDL, increased triglycerides, and increased blood sugars.

For these reasons, the **Track Your Plaque** approach does not dictate a specific percent fat restriction but is a practical approach based on several important principles. Following these principles in your food selection will, in effect, cause you to be on a diet that is moderately low-fat and moderately low in carbohydrate, but these are secondary concerns. (If you insist on knowing the constitution of the typical diet constructed from these principles, it is generally a 24–30% fat diet, a level of fat intake that allows the best balance of benefits without adverse effects on lipid/lipoprotein parameters.)

Will I lose weight?

Don't confuse diets for weight-loss with diets for reduction of heart disease risk. The popular media often confuse the two. Losing weight can indeed reduce risk for heart disease. A diet that provides a rational, comprehensive approach to heart disease prevention should be much more than that. The Atkin's diet provides a good example. Patients often ask if they should begin an Atkins' diet for their heart. But the Atkins' diet (at least the so-called "induction phase") is an effective tool for weight-loss. It is not, in my view, a healthy means to reduce heart disease risk (beyond weight-loss effects). The high saturated fat content, the lack of fiber, flavonoids, and phytonutrients, I believe, lead to heightened risk of cancer, osteoporosis, kidney stones, and bladder infections if followed for more than a few months, though you may lose 10 or more pounds. This doesn't make sense. I don't think it's much different than telling you to start smoking to lose weight—it works, but it's clearly not very healthy.

The **Track Your Plaque** nutrition principles do promote weight-loss. The majority of participants in the program enjoy an abrupt initial drop of 10–20 lbs. in the first three months, followed by a gradual downward trend in weight over the ensuing year. Losing excess weight can indeed significantly impact on your lipid and lipoprotein patterns, reduce a hidden diabetic tendency, and simply make you feel better, all of which contribute to control over plaque. Following the nutrition principles here will achieve *more* than weight-loss.

Can medicines make up for a bad diet?

Just how important is diet? Some people ask, "What if I follow only *part* of the program? I'll take the medicines and supplements and exercise, but I really don't want to give up my steaks, bacon, butter, cupcakes, and chips. Can I still reduce my score?"

People who eat this way do not enjoy the kind of control over their coronary plaque as people who pay close attention to diet. For one thing, eating an average American diet virtually ensures excessive weight gain. When you ingest large quantities of saturated fat and refined starches, many lipid/lipoprotein abnormalities (particularly HDL, LDL particle size, and VLDL) become more difficult to control, necessitating more and more medicines and ultimately causing growth of coronary plaque. There are also aspects of diet that cannot be controlled by any medication or supplement. For instance, post-prandial hyperlipemia, or the after-meal flood of fat in the blood that occurs the first few hours after eating, is largely influenced by the fat content of your diet. It does not respond well to any specific treatment, so that the foods you choose are crucial determinants of whether you will or will not shower your arteries with globules of fat for the eight or so hours after a meal.

I cured myself of heart disease with a low-fat diet!

So declared Sandy L., a 49-year-old secretary. Because her mother's family was plagued with heart disease, Sandy had undergone a heart scan one year earlier. Her score: 51, a score that put her in the 90th percentile, a worrisome score for a young woman. But Sandy had strong feelings against the medicines and supplements that we discussed when five different lipoprotein abnormalities were diagnosed causing her coronary plaque.

Sandy was determined to deal with her coronary disease with diet alone. She followed a very strict vegetarian diet free of saturated and hydrogenated oils, essentially no flour containing baked products or sweets, and concentrated on vegetables, fruits, and whole grains-an excellent diet. Her lipoprotein patterns improved modestly but were far from fully corrected, but she continued to resist the idea of any other treatments.

To assess her results, I asked Sandy to have another heart scan 18 months later. This time, her score was 98—*a near-doubling*. With this indisputable proof of progressive plaque growth, Sandy finally agreed to accept the recommended treatments for her lipoprotein disorders.

The lesson: diet is important, but even a near perfect effort can not cure you of rapidly growing coronary plaque.

How do I know my diet is working?

Lipids and lipoproteins can be used to gauge your success through diet. For instance, let's say you have a low HDL, excessive small LDL, and a high triglyceride level identified at the start of your program. You make changes in diet, increase physical activity, and lose 20 pounds. You also begin niacin along with some other treatments to correct your lipoprotein patterns. Is that good enough?

This can be decided by reassessing lipids or lipoproteins to see whether your abnormalities have been corrected. (**Track Your Plaque** lipid and lipoprotein endpoints are listed in chapter 8.) But don't commit the mistake that some people make. They succeed in making lifestyle changes, then declare, "I've stopped all my medicines and supplements since I'm doing so well!" Unfortunately, just feeling good or losing 20 pounds are *not* reliable indications of whether your genetic lipid/lipoprotein patterns have been corrected. That decision can only be made by repeating lipid or lipoprotein testing and, ultimately, by the effects on your heart scan score.

Let's now discuss the six **Track Your Plaque** principles of healthy eating.

Principle No. 1: Low-fat, good fat

Despite mixed results with ultra-low-fat diets, restricting fat intake to a moderate degree is still a healthy strategy. While we need fat for regeneration of tissues, energy, brain function, etc., we do not want to provide the ingredients to grow coronary plaque. The key is to eliminate two kinds of fats as completely as possible from your diet: saturated and hydrogenated.

Fats that are saturated have all the hydrogen atoms they can accommodate, i.e., they are "saturated" with hydrogen. Saturated fats are solid at room temperature, like the fat on Porterhouse steak or vegetable shortening. *All foods you eat should be low in saturated fat.* Saturated fats serve no good purpose whatsoever and are entirely unnecessary for health. Do away with saturated fat completely and you'll be better off. Your goal should be as close to zero grams of saturated fat per day as possible. This means minimizing, or even eliminating, fried foods, sausage, bacon, egg yolks, butter and other full-fat dairy products like cheese. When you choose red meats, they should be lean as possible with the excess fat trimmed and oil drained during cooking. The saturated fats in these foods raise LDL cholesterol and LDL particle number/apoprotein B, are rich in empty calories, increase blood pressure, and increase risk of cancer.

Vegetables and fruits are low in saturated fat, as are chicken (with the skin removed), fish, raw nuts, egg whites (or "Egg Beaters"), and low or non-fat dairy products. While red meats can be a significant source of saturated fat, smaller portions (four ounces) of lean cuts with the oil drained off eaten once or twice per week leaves you within safe bounds. Alternatively, game meat, like venison or buffalo, can be a low saturated fat source of red meat.

The other fat to avoid is *hydrogenated* fat. Hydrogenated fats are synthetic products found in many if not most processed foods because manufacturers put them there. In this twentieth century method of processing, oils are heated to high temperatures while hydrogen gas is bubbled through, yielding a mixture of oils that contain extra hydrogen molecules in an unnatural "trans" (opposite sides of a carbon chain) configuration. (Naturally occurring oils are in a "cis" configuration, with hydrogens on the same side, which makes them liquid at room temperature.) Two common examples of hydrogenated fats are margarine and vegetable shortening. Trans-fatty acids created by hydrogenation help add body to processed foods and extend shelf-life. For these reasons, food manufacturers love to add hydrogenated oils to cookies and cakes, pies, pastries, all sorts of snack chips, frozen foods, salad dressings and mayonnaise, and many convenience foods. Stick margarines are higher in hydrogenated fats than tub margarines, since hydrogenation is required for solidity. As public demand for convenience and indulgence grows, food manufacturers have obliged by creating more highly processed foods that taste and look "better" with hydrogenated oils.

Hydrogenated fats are *worse* than saturated fats. They not only raise LDL cholesterol, but also lower HDL cholesterol. They can also increase the dreaded Lp(a). Pay particular attention to your hydrogenated fat intake if your LDL is greater than 100 mg/dl, if your HDL is <60 mg/dl, or if your Lp(a) is elevated. Unfortunately, manufacturers are not presently required to specify the quantity of hydrogenated fats or trans-fatty acids on product labels. (They will be required to do so by the FDA in the near future.) You will therefore have to rely on the list of ingredients. If "hydrogenated oil" or "partially hydrogenated oil" is listed, avoid it.

Hydrogenated oils are bad news beyond issues of cholesterol and are being increasingly implicated in other disease conditions. Nutrition scientists have observed disturbing phenomena in cells incorporating hydrogenated fatty acids into their structure: Fluidity of cell membranes becomes abnormal, signal processing is distorted, and internal cell reactions are disturbed. We'll likely be hearing more in future about how hydrogenation is related to cancer.

Polyunsaturated fats are a mixed bag. Most vegetable oils (non-hydrogenated) are rich in *omega-6* fatty acids. Polyunsaturated means that the structure of the fatty acids have many double bonds and are thus unsaturated in hydrogen atoms. "Omega-6" refers to a double bond at the sixth position in the carbon chain. Corn, safflower, sunflower, palm, and soybean oils contain abundant omega-6 fatty acids. Polyunsaturation makes these oils liquids at room temperature. Approximately 14% of the fatty acids in these oils are saturated, also. Compared to saturated fats from animal sources, omega-6 polyunsaturated oils do not raise LDL cholesterol, and may lower it a tiny amount. Polyunsaturated oils should be viewed as neutral, that is, neither terribly damaging nor terribly beneficial. These oils are acceptable for use in cooking and in foods, but are best used sparingly. There are better forms of oils to use that provide benefit rather than a neutral effect but with identical calorie content. Remember that oils are very calorie dense, with nine calories per gram (compared to four calories per gram for both proteins and carbohydrates). One tablespoon of any oil, good or bad, contains 14 grams of fat, or 126 calories.

Now the good...

In sharp contrast, *omega-3* polyunsaturated fats, with a double bond located at the third carbon atom rather than the sixth, are a world apart from other fats. A large amount of evidence argues that, if there are good fats, it's the omega-3s. Omega-3 fatty acids are so beneficial that they can be used as a treatment, as well as a preventive strategy.

The two primary omega-3 fatty acids are docosahexaenoic acid, or DHA, and eicosapentaenoic acid, or EPA. Omega-3s were first suspected to provide heart benefits when epidemiologists tried to understand why Eskimos, despite a diet rich in fat, suffered few heart attacks. Eskimos feast on cold-water fish containing large quantities of omega-3 fatty acids. (Omega-3s prevent fish cell membranes from solidifying in cold water.) Subsequent studies have bolstered the argument that omega-3 fatty acids are the component of diet in fish eating cultures responsible for reducing the number of heart attacks.

Omega-3s lower blood pressure, lower triglycerides, raise HDL (a little bit), and make LDL particles bigger. Several large studies have shown that when people who've suffered heart attacks eat a diet rich in omega-3s or take fish oil supplements, the risk of dying of heart attack is slashed by 30–40%.

Omega-3s provide benefits outside the heart, too. Evidence suggests that they have cancer preventing effects, may inhibit the appearance of Alzheimer's dementia, and have even been used with some success in treating depression.

Fish are the principal source for omega-3 fatty acids: cod, halibut, trout, salmon, mackerel, tuna, sardines, but not shellfish. A large study in Chicago workers showed that just eating two servings of fish a month was enough to sharply drop the risk of dying of heart attack. Of course, we are looking for benefits beyond just avoiding heart attack—we want to reduce the growth of coronary plaque. For this purpose, the use of fish oil supplements is necessary, a means of ensuring higher intakes of omega-3s. It is generally impractical to obtain the quantity necessary for our purposes through diet. (You would have to eat three to five servings of fish per day to achieve therapeutic doses.) We will discuss later how to use fish oil supplements in your personal **Track Your Plaque** program. It is still worth including fish in your diet as often as possible, at least once or twice per week. Obviously, fish should be baked, not fried.

Flaxseed oil is another source of omega-3s. However, the omega-3s in flaxseed oil don't occur as DHA or EPA, but as linolenic acid, another fatty acid. Flaxseed oil is nearly tasteless and is easier to take than foul smelling fish oil. But the conversion of linolenic acid to the active DHA/EPA is inefficient, about one part DHA/EPA for every 10 parts linolenic acid taken, and a huge dose of flaxseed oil is therefore required to reproduce the lipid/lipoprotein benefits of fish oil (especially triglyceride and VLDL reduction). Because the data with fish sources of omega-3s are much more persuasive, fish oil is the preferred source. Flaxseed remains a second choice after fish oil. (Flaxseed oil is better as a food than as a supplement. Unfortunately, it is expensive, often costing around $8–10 for a 12 oz bottle. If you can afford the expense, use flaxseed oil for cooking or salad oil, and you will be using the most abundant omega-3-containing vegetable oil available.)

Omega-3 fatty acids in fish oil are more than preventive agents. They can also be used to treat specific lipid and lipoprotein abnormalities. The therapeutic uses of omega-3 fatty acids are simply an exaggeration of the preventive effects. Much of fish oil's benefit stems from its triglyceride lowering effect (about 30% reduction, occasionally up to 50%). A reduction in triglycerides triggers a domino effect of reduced VLDL, which thereby reduces small LDL and raises HDL. Fish oil also lowers the amount of fibrinogen in your blood, as well as reducing lipoprotein (a) a modest degree.

The other healthy group of oils are the *monounsaturated* fatty acids (mono = one double bond and not fully bound with hydrogen). Monounsaturates are gaining attention lately due to the success of the Mediterranean diet in reducing risk of heart attack. The Lyon Heart Study examined the health benefits of a Mediterranean diet rich in olive oil, vegetables, and fish, similar to that eaten along the Mediterranean coast in Europe. People following this diet (as compared to a more American like diet of red meat, fast and processed foods, etc.) suffered 40% fewer heart attacks.

The monounsaturates are preferable to the polyunsaturates. They are certainly better than saturated fats, and so foods rich in monounsaturated oils can make healthy substitutes for both saturated and polyunsaturated fat. Using modest quantities of olive oil (extra virgin, cold-pressed) or canola oil, both of which are rich in monounsaturated forms, is safe and healthy. When you need oil for your salad dressing or cooking, reach for olive or canola, rather than corn or mixed vegetable oils. Olive and canola oils are also somewhat lower in saturated fats. (Remember that *all* oils are calorie dense, even the omega-3s and monounsaturated.)

Raw nuts are a great source of monounsaturated fats, especially raw almonds and walnuts. People are often afraid to eat nuts because of their high-fat content. But most of the fat is monounsaturated. Raw nuts are filling, requiring many hours to digest, and eliminate craving for snacks and sweets. In fact, eating ¼–½ cup of raw almonds or walnuts every day can lower cholesterol by 10–15%. Just watch out for the calories if you exceed this quantity.

How important are fat grams?

If you gravitate towards oils and foods rich in omega-3 and monounsaturated fatty acids and thereby eliminate the LDL raising effect of fats, then the only adverse effect of fat in your diet is excessive calories. Let me re-phrase that idea: Remove the saturated and the hydrogenated fats from your diet and minimize the polyunsaturated fats, and replace them with omega-3 and monounsaturated fats, *and the LDL raising effect of fats is gone.*

Too much of a good thing can be bad. Can you gain weight by eating too many raw nuts, using too much canola oil in your salad dressing and olive oil in your tomato sauce? Of course you can. The average American daily diet of unrestricted fat commonly contains 110–120 grams of fat, or 990–1080 calories per day from fat. That's just under half your daily calories from fat. Proponents of low-fat diets have argued that the high caloric density of fat should be replaced by the low caloric density of protein and carbohydrates (four calories per gram). For example, replacing the 110 grams fat with 110 grams of carbohydrate would yield 440 calories, or 550 calories less than an equal weight in fat.

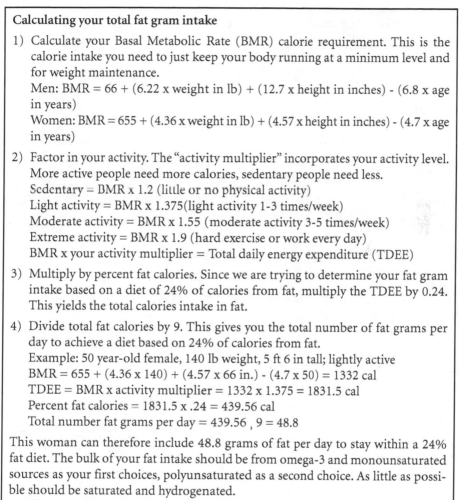

Calculating your total fat gram intake

1) Calculate your Basal Metabolic Rate (BMR) calorie requirement. This is the calorie intake you need to just keep your body running at a minimum level and for weight maintenance.

   Men: BMR = 66 + (6.22 x weight in lb) + (12.7 x height in inches) - (6.8 x age in years)

   Women: BMR = 655 + (4.36 x weight in lb) + (4.57 x height in inches) - (4.7 x age in years)

2) Factor in your activity. The "activity multiplier" incorporates your activity level. More active people need more calories, sedentary people need less.

   Sedentary = BMR x 1.2 (little or no physical activity)

   Light activity = BMR x 1.375(light activity 1-3 times/week)

   Moderate activity = BMR x 1.55 (moderate activity 3-5 times/week)

   Extreme activity = BMR x 1.9 (hard exercise or work every day)

   BMR x your activity multiplier = Total daily energy expenditure (TDEE)

3) Multiply by percent fat calories. Since we are trying to determine your fat gram intake based on a diet of 24% of calories from fat, multiply the TDEE by 0.24. This yields the total calories intake in fat.

4) Divide total fat calories by 9. This gives you the total number of fat grams per day to achieve a diet based on 24% of calories from fat.

   Example: 50 year-old female, 140 lb weight, 5 ft 6 in tall; lightly active

   BMR = 655 + (4.36 x 140) + (4.57 x 66 in.) - (4.7 x 50) = 1332 cal

   TDEE = BMR x activity multiplier = 1332 x 1.375 = 1831.5 cal

   Percent fat calories = 1831.5 x .24 = 439.56 cal

   Total number fat grams per day = 439.56 , 9 = 48.8

This woman can therefore include 48.8 grams of fat per day to stay within a 24% fat diet. The bulk of your fat intake should be from omega-3 and monounsaturated sources as your first choices, polyunsaturated as a second choice. As little as possible should be saturated and hydrogenated.

If your goal is weight-loss, you should adjust your total intake of calories to fall below that of your total daily energy expenditure. This will reduce your allowed fat gram intake accordingly.

There's some merit to this argument. Let's face it: the average American is overweight and needs to cut calorie intake. Most people can easily reduce the amount of calories in their diet by shaving off the excess half of fat intake. The downside of this argument is that, if too many fat calories are eliminated, they're often replaced by calories from carbohydrates. This results in increased insulin and blood sugar levels, a drop in HDL, and increase in triglycerides. Additional undesirable effects in lipoprotein particle size develop. Dr. Ronald

Krauss of Stanford has shown that many people who begin with normal LDL particle size will develop the undesirable small particles when fat intake drops below 20% of calories. (Recall that the ultra-low-fat diets are usually 10% fat.) These people may actually *increase* their risk of heart disease.

If your diet is weighed heavily in favor of omega-3 and monounsaturated fats, *then the only reason to count total fat grams is to limit calories.* The great majority of people therefore do better, both from a lipid as well as a weight control perspective, on a 24% fat intake. The calories from fat are nearly cut in half compared to an unrestricted diet. Since most of us are unable to think about fat intake on a percentage of calories basis, you can count fat grams instead. For the average 5 foot 10 inch, 50-year old man weighing 180 pounds who is moderately active (exercising three to five times per week), the daily caloric intake is 2688 calories. The expected fat gram intake for a man this size would be 72 grams. The average 5 foot 5 inch, 50-year old woman weighing 130 pounds who is also moderately active should take in around 1989 calories. This translates into 53 grams of fat per day. To calculate your calorie and fat gram intake based on sex, height, and activity level, see the accompanying table. (These calorie intakes are for weight *maintenance*, not weight-loss.)

This approach to fat intake management is easy to follow. It allows many delicious, filling dishes, since there is plenty of room to use healthy oils like olive oil and canola oil-based margarines. You enjoy the LDL lowering benefits of a low-fat diet, but avoid the negative effects of an excessive restriction. Lean protein sources like baked chicken and fish can easily fit into this regimen, as can flaxseed products, raw nuts, and other healthy oil sources of omega-3 and monounsaturated fatty acids. If weight-loss is among your interests, this approach combined with the other **Track Your Plaque** nutrition principles generally leads to a gradual, sustained drop in excess weight. (We will discuss weight-loss more thoroughly in chapter 10.)

Principle No. 2: Foods should be rich in fiber

There's a lot more healthy punch to fiber than making you regular. Fiber is a great nutritional tool that's inexpensive and provides an array of lipid/lipoprotein benefits.

Foods contain two different types of fiber: soluble and insoluble. Bran, as in bran cereal and whole wheat bread, is a common source of *insoluble* fiber, the indigestible portion of the grain removed during food-manufacturing processes. Insoluble fiber increases stool bulk and thereby reduces the risk of colon cancer. Insoluble fiber can also lower blood pressure to a modest degree. People who include abundant quantities of unrefined, insoluble fiber-rich foods in their diet are healthier, tend to be less overweight, and live longer. Good sources of insoluble fiber include whole grain products, wild rice, vegetables, and fruits. Processed foods, especially white flour products, are very low in insoluble fiber.

Soluble fiber is so-called because, when it comes into contact with water, becomes gel-like. As a gel, water saturated soluble fiber binds cholesterol and fat in the intestine, which then passes in your stool. Soluble fiber is a great natural way to reduce your LDL cholesterol and LDL particle number/apoprotein B. You'll find soluble fiber in starchy beans—lima, pinto, Spanish, black, red, soy, kidney, etc.; oatmeal and oat bran (as beta-glucan); berries; and apples, applesauce, and citrus rinds (as pectin). One cup of kidney beans a day (containing 5.0 grams of soluble fiber), for example, can lower LDL cholesterol by 10–15%.

You can tally up your fiber gram count to get a sense for your daily fiber intake. The FDA requires food manufacturers to list the total content of fiber on labels, though specifically listing soluble fiber content is optional. Most Americans, with highly-refined, high-fat, high sugar diets, take in a meager 14 grams of total fiber per day. Your goal should be a total fiber intake (soluble+insoluble) of *no less than* 35 grams per day. If you have a high LDL cholesterol or LDL particle number/apoprotein B, you might try to weigh your fiber intake more heavily in favor of soluble fiber foods, and achieve an even greater total fiber intake, as high as 50+ grams. A rough rule of thumb is that, for every additional one gram of soluble fiber intake, you can lower your total cholesterol by one to two points.

If counting fiber grams is impractical for you, try following several basic guidelines that stack your diet full of healthy fibers:

- Always choose unrefined foods over refined, e.g., whole grain bread (whole *grain* is better than whole *wheat*, especially if oats are among the primary ingredients of the whole grain), not white; whole wheat pasta, not white; brown or wild rice, not white.

Rich Sources of Soluble Fiber	
Oat bran (1/3 cup, uncooked)	*2.0 g*
Oatmeal (1 cup, cooked)	*1.9 g*
Kidney beans (1 cup, cooked)	*5.0 g*
Pinto beans (1 cup, cooked)	*4.6 g*
Lentils (1 cup, cooked)	*3.4 g*
Peas (1 cup, cooked)	*5.4 g*
Sweet potato (1 baked)	1.3 g
White potato (1 baked)	0.9 g
Broccoli (1 cup, cooked)	1.8 g
Prunes (4)	1.9 g
Pear (1)	1.1 g
Apple (1)	0.9 g
Blueberries (1/2 cup)	2.0 g

The foods highlighted above are great sources of soluble fiber. Compare this to the soluble fiber content of whole wheat bread, which has 0.5 g soluble fiber in two slices.

- Add soluble fiber sources such as flaxseed or oat bran to yogurt, fruit smoothies, cereals, salads, casseroles, etc.
- Try to include at least one half cup serving of beans in one meal every day.
- Use whole berries—strawberries, blueberries, blackberries, raspberries, cranberries—whenever possible.
- Sprinkle raw seeds and nuts on salads, yogurt, and cereals, or, even better, eat them plain. Best are raw sunflower and pumpkin seeds, raw almonds, walnuts, and pecans. They're loaded with insoluble fiber.
- Eat vegetables raw whenever possible. Some fiber is broken down into simpler carbohydrate components when cooked.
- Eat the skin or peel. In apples, pears, citrus fruits, cucumbers, eggplant, etc., much of the fiber and the phytonutrients are in the skin. Wash first, of course. With citrus fruits, you don't need to eat the entire rind but just the white portion for its pectin.

In addition to LDL lowering effects, fiber smoothes out spikes in blood sugar that carbohydrates cause. This reduces triglycerides and even blocks the development of diabetes. Loading up on fiber sources also helps lose weight, as you feel satisfied after a meal. Fiber-rich foods are very slowly digested and the blunted post-prandial sugar curve delays the trigger to eat again.

Combining several fiber strategies and increasing your daily fiber intake to 35 gm or greater can drop your LDL, apoprotein B, or LDL particle number up to 18–20%. That's nearly as good as the cholesterol lowering drugs.

You can probably see that fiber is found most abundantly in whole, unprocessed foods. Processing by food manufacturers very commonly involves removal of much of the fiber content. This leads us to Principle No. 3.

Principle No. 3: Foods should be *unprocessed* and *unrefined*

Principle number 3 is closely related to Principle number 2. In general, unprocessed foods are also fiber-rich foods. But there's a lot more to this issue.

Unprocessed foods are *whole* foods—the bran is not removed (as in white flour and white rice), not dried (like instant oatmeal and instant mashed potatoes), not powdered (cocoa, instant soups, sauces), and not a mix (pancake and cake mixes, macaroni and cheese). Unprocessed foods *do not require reconstitution*—adding water and heating, or some similar process. Unprocessed foods are not modified by hydrogenation, desiccation, are not sweetened and don't contain artificial flavorings or colorings.

Unprocessed foods tend to look just as they occur naturally. You may have to remove an outer shell (nuts) or skin (oranges, avocados) but they remain essentially intact. Of course, you may need to cut whole foods into smaller pieces, but the basic structure remains the same. Unprocessed foods are generally fresh, although canned and frozen forms are acceptable since no significant nutritive value is lost with these forms of processing. When food is left whole, it retains more of its original, naturally occurring nutrients. It is also digested more slowly, causing a gradual rise in blood sugar. Diabetics who switch to a diet of unprocessed foods commonly experience dramatic drops in blood sugar, often sufficient to reduce requirements for medication or insulin. (This applies to type II, or non-insulin dependent, diabetics only, and not type I, or insulin-dependent diabetics.)

Unprocessed foods lower blood pressure. The fiber and phytonutrients (naturally occurring plant nutrients) provide a blood pressure lowering effect absent from processed foods. Most people who switch from a processed to an unprocessed diet enjoy a drop of 5–10 mg Hg drop in blood pressure within a few weeks to months.

Unprocessed foods are also often very colorful foods. Look at the wonderfully deep colors of plums, eggplant, oranges, tomatoes, and spinach. Colorful foods are rich in flavonoids, naturally occurring substances that provide a broad range of health benefits. From a heart disease perspective, flavonoids lower LDL cholesterol and raise HDL slightly, provide an anti-oxidant function that makes LDL less harmful, lower blood pressure, block abnormal clotting by platelets, block adhesion of inflammatory blood cells to plaque, and may reduce risk of heart attack. The scientific data documenting the benefits of flavonoid-rich foods are growing rapidly. Besides deeply colored fruits and vegetables, olive oil (extra virgin only), grape seed oil, green tea and red wines are also plentiful sources of healthful flavonoids. Incidentally, of the various components of grapes (pulp, seeds, and skin) the seeds contain 60–70% of the flavonoid content of the entire grape. For this reason, red wine and grape juice (both of which retain much of the flavonoid content of the seed) and whole grapes eaten with the seeds can be especially good for you.

The growing appreciation of the power of flavonoids has caused many people to speculate whether taking a pill concentrate of one or more flavonoids might heighten benefits. However, of the many thousands of naturally occurring flavonoids, *combinations* of many flavonoids seem to work better than taking just one or a few. Once again, benefits of the whole food seem to win over that of processed derivatives. Much work needs to be done in living humans to validate these suggestive data, but the whole concept of flavonoids is worth watching over the next 10 years. In the meantime, a diet rich in deeply colored, whole vegetables and fruits is unquestionably worth following.

What makes processed foods so undesirable? The various forms of processing used by manufacturers are designed for taste and convenience. When components like bran are removed from grain products, a source of B vitamins and fiber (soluble and insoluble) is discarded. The process of desiccation destroys many of the heat sensitive phytonutrients. It also raises glycemic index (see Principle No. 5); after ingestion, you experience a sharp rise in blood sugar followed by an abrupt and exaggerated fall. Foods with high glycemic index also lower HDL, raise triglycerides, and can unmask a latent diabetic tendency. It can also play havoc with your mood and energy and cause weight gain.

Processing also frequently involves undesirable additives that can have negative effects on your health. Additives are intended to improve taste, consistency, or extend shelf-life. They include hydrogenated oils, food colorings, sweeteners like corn syrup and sugar, and preservatives. They make food look prettier, last longer, and maintain texture and consistency during storage, but they do your body little good. The hydrogenated oil and trans-fatty acids in many baked products (cakes, cookies, chips) and margarine raise LDL cholesterol and LDL particle number/apoprotein B and lower HDL. High fructose corn syrup (discussed further below) is a sweetener that kids love and is found in everything from fruit drinks to spaghetti sauce. High fructose corn syrup raises triglycerides up to 30%. Increased triglycerides can contribute to many undesirable lipoprotein patterns, like small LDL and excess VLDL, and may even increase the likelihood of diabetes.

Unprocessed foods are not glamorous. They are rarely featured by advertisers. They don't generally have fancy labels or packaging—you might even have to buy them "bulk". Think about this for a moment. Just about all the advertising you see for food products involves highly processed foods: cereals, soft drinks, frozen, dried/desiccated, instant, reconstituted, etc. Watch daytime TV some afternoon and you'll see a powerful demonstration of this. You won't see ads promoting green peppers or flaxseed. The expensive, clever, sexy advertising is reserved for higher profit margin processed foods. I was watching Saturday morning cartoons with my kids recently when a gripping, visually irresistible commercial came on, accompanied by wild, foot tapping music. We couldn't take our eyes off the TV until the closing shot: an ad for macaroni and cheese (ingredients: processed white flour, dried cheese, hydrogenated oils—garbage, in short). That's a lot of expense and effort for a nutritionally empty product.

The temptations of processed foods are all around us. Imagine the reaction of a hungry inhabitant of a third world nation on walking the aisles of the supermarkets we have in this country. Shelf after shelf, aisle after aisle of eye-catching, colorful, enticing processed foods. Not one or two kinds of cookies and cupcakes to choose from, but hundreds! I'll bet that you and your family have sampled (or indulged to excess) in most of them. The temptations are tremendous.

I stress this issue because many people struggle when forced to part with the glitz and glamour of processed foods. The marketing people who create these ads are very clever. They know that advertising can make you feel good about eating a certain food. They want you to feel proud to feed your family a "healthy" dish, sexy if you drink a certain drink, successful if you can whip up a dinner of convenience foods in five minutes.

If sugar is bad, high fructose corn syrup is worse!

High fructose corn syrup (corn syrup highly enriched in fructose) is hard to escape. It is a major ingredient in all sorts of processed foods. You'll find it in soft drinks, pancake syrups, sweet breakfast cereals, candies, and sweetened yogurts. You'll also find it in less obvious places like bread, low-fat salad dressings, tomato sauces, ketchup, and even beer. Americans consume more high fructose corn syrup than ever before, an average of nearly 65 lbs per year (compared to < 1 lb in 1970).

High fructose corn syrup is sweeter than sugar. Manufacturers love it because it's cheap, has a long shelf-life, and even has anti-bacterial properties (so foods won't spoil easily). Kids especially love the extra sweetness and, when permitted, will gobble down huge quantities of fructose containing products.

High fructose corn syrup is not a problem because of glycemic index, but brings a whole new collection of troubles. Unlike table sugar (sucrose), high fructose corn syrup appears to provoke several alarming health effects:

1. A significant increase in *triglycerides—Often 50% or more.*

2. *No suppression of appetite.* In other words, when you ingest ordinary sugar, appetite eventually is suppressed. High fructose corn syrup does not stimulate the release of the appetite suppressing hormone, *leptin.* Your craving for more sweets and food is therefore not turned-off.

3. *No insulin response.* Sugar provokes insulin release; high fructose corn syrup does not. This leads to abnormal liver responses, including manufacturing more triglycerides. This can lead to a greater likelihood of weight gain and diabetes.

Some critics are blaming high fructose corn syrup for the growing epidemic of obesity in adults and children. This product is finding its way into more and more products, while the average American is consuming greater and greater quantities.

How can you avoid this ubiquitous product? Check the label: if high fructose corn syrup is listed, particularly as one of the first ingredients, then you should avoid it. You will discover high fructose corn syrup in many seemingly "healthy" products like low-fat salad dressings. Even better, follow the **Track Your Plaque** principle of avoiding processed foods and selecting only whole, unprocessed foods. This strategy alone will help you drastically reduce your intake of this terrible product.

You'll get *none* of this reinforcement when you restrict yourself to the world of unprocessed foods. You'll feel like a burlap sack in a shop full of Gucci handbags. Yet it's the unprocessed, unrefined foods that are powerful tools for your health.

When you go to the grocery store, notice how the products are arranged. In most major supermarkets, unprocessed foods are grouped around the periphery; the processed foods in the central aisles. Use this layout to your advantage. Shop all you can at the edges where you'll find vegetables, fruits, and dairy products. Avoid the inner sections as much as possible. Try this a few times, and you will notice how truly unnecessary the products in the central aisles really are. Except for cleaning products and the occasional condiment like mustard or seasonings, you can do practically all your shopping in the outer aisles. You will avoid the white flour baked products, cakes, pies, donuts, cookies, white pastas, dry packaged foods, candies, soft drinks, chips, etc. You will sacrifice convenience but you will gain health.

If you need some confirmation of the detrimental

How to increase your insulin sensitivity

If you have adult-onset (type II) diabetes or borderline diabetes, does this mean you have a deficiency of insulin in your blood?

No. Ninety percent of the time it means that you have *too much* insulin, but your body's cells have become *resistant* to insulin. Blood sugar goes up, since sugar is unable to enter cells. One approach that may help is to increase your body's insulin sensitivity, your body's ability to respond to its own insulin. Life habits or supplements that increase insulin sensitivity include:

- Exercise—with a focus on *duration* (at least 30 minutes per session), *not intensity*. The longer and more frequent, the better. Try to include strength training, which *really* helps.
- Weight-loss (if overweight)—a dramatic effect that may even convert a recent diabetic to a non-diabetic.
- Omega-3 fatty acids—though only a modest effect. Omega-3s probably work by reducing release of fatty acids in the blood.
- Chromium supplements—e.g., chromium picolinate 200-800 mcg per day has in some studies improved blood sugars by increasing insulin's effects. The effect tends to be modest.
- Sleep. Chronic lack of a full night's sleep can antagonize insulin's effects. This can be a powerful phenomenon and is very common. Catching up on lost sleep to payback your "sleep deficit" can require up to three weeks of sleeping eight to ten hours per night.
- Raw nuts, oat bran, lean proteins, healthy fats. All work by slowing the absorption of sugar into the blood, which over time leads to increased insulin sensitivity. Adding any of these foods to high glycemic index foods can partially suppress the initial blood sugar spike.

If you don't have blood sugar problems but have a low HDL(<40 mg/dl), high triglycerides (>150 mg/dl), small LDL or excessive VLDL, this advice applies to you, as well, since these are frequently markers for a hidden genetic diabetic tendency.

effects of eating a diet filled with processed foods, try this experiment. While you're standing in the check-out line at the grocery store, notice who is overweight, then take notice of the foods they are buying. You will likely observe that shoppers who struggle with their weight have shopping carts full of instant, powdered, hydrogenated, baked, sugar coated, etc. foods. Conversely, thin, fit shoppers generally have carts predominantly full of produce.

If the avoidance of processed foods becomes a guiding principle of your diet, you will enjoy many benefits that can minimize your need for medications to treat your lipoprotein abnormalities, blood pressure, and diabetes. Of course, some processed foods are a practical necessity in our lives. You and I aren't going to crush tomatoes to make our own ketchup or press our own olive oil. If you adhere to this basic rule in most of what you eat, you'll enjoy huge positive healthy changes.

Principle No. 4: Foods should have a *low glycemic index*

Let's say you ate a meal and then measured your blood sugar every 15 minutes afterwards, while the food was digested and absorbed. You'd observe that some foods cause a rapid, high rise in blood sugar, others cause a slow, gradual rise. You can then compare these patterns to white sugar or white bread as a reference (since they yield the most dramatic spike in blood sugar). This measure is called "glycemic index." Put simply, foods with a low glycemic index cause a slow, gradual rise in blood sugar after ingestion. These tend to be protein and fat containing foods. Carbohydrates have a high glycemic index. Initial exaggerated rises in sugar often then plummet to below normal, thus the hypoglycemic symptoms of shakiness, mental fogginess, and fatigue some people experience an hour or two after a high glycemic index meal. Candies, cookies, soft drinks, white bread, white flour pasta, and potatoes (all carbohydrates) have a high glycemic index. Processed foods that are sweetened with sugar virtually always provoke an exaggerated glycemic response, as well. Vegetables, meats, dairy products and nuts, on the other hand,—all non-carbohydrate foods—have low glycemic indexes. The glycemic index of the American diet has climbed higher and higher over the past four decades as our relative intake of carbohydrates increases and we reach for more highly processed foods.

Unprocessed foods are higher in fiber and have lower glycemic indexes, as complex fibers slow digestion and release of sugars. Processed foods with fiber removed—instant rice, white bread and other white flour baked products, and sugary cereals—all raise your blood sugar just as if you were dipping your spoon straight into the sugar bowl.

Why is this important? With high glycemic index foods, sugar is absorbed rapidly, provoking a large insulin release. Excessive insulin causes hypoglycemia, or low blood sugar. Hypoglycemia is a potent trigger to eat again to compensate for the drop in sugar levels, and provokes *hyperphagia*, or over-eating. People experiencing this effect will reflexively crave refined carbohydrates, because of the rapid relief they provide for the drop in blood sugar. The stage is then set for a cycle of hypoglycemia and overeating that leads to weight gain and diabetes.

High insulin levels also trigger a complex chain of events that results in a drop in HDL cholesterol and a rise in triglycerides. Triglycerides can reach very high levels of several hundred or higher. The increased availability of triglycerides creates triglyceride rich particles, such as VLDL and small LDL. These, of course, are the particles that make coronary plaque grow.

Low glycemic index foods do not result in high blood sugars, excessive insulin, hypoglycemia, hyperphagia, and the weight gain caused by high glycemic index foods. Low glycemic index foods also don't create undesirable lipoproteins like small LDL and VLDL and are therefore less likely to promote growth of coronary plaque. What's more, low glycemic index foods, since they are more slowly digested and metabolized, are more filling, making you less apt to indulge in snacks.

Does this mean that you should totally shun foods that have a high glycemic index? No, it simply means that you should *favor* low vs. high index foods. For instance, avoid highly processed breakfast cereals made of puffed wheat or corn flakes (high glycemic index) and consider replacing with low-fat yogurt garnished with sliced peaches, raisins, and raw nuts (all low glycemic index), or an oat based granola sweetened with honey and fruit. Some foods are so offensive in this regard that you should only rarely indulge in them: soft drinks, white flour baked products like cakes and cookies, snack chips, breakfast drinks, and candy. Fruit juices, though they contain many desirable ingredients, still evoke the exaggerated blood sugar response and should therefore be minimized. Please refer to the accompanying table for relative indexes for some common foods. Try to choose those foods that fall into the low or intermediate glycemic index categories. At those times you do eat foods with a high glycemic index, consider eating raw nuts or adding oat bran, flaxseed, or other fibers to blunt the rise in sugars.

Breakfast, in particular, can be a high glycemic index landmine. You'll eliminate many high glycemic index foods in your diet just by concentrating on selecting low glycemic index foods for breakfast: low-fat yogurt (watch the sweeteners, often containing high fructose corn syrup), cottage cheese, egg whites, oat bran cereal, fruits (except bananas), oat-based granolas (buy brands without added sugar), and raw nuts and seeds, either by themselves or mixed with other foods.

If you have a low HDL (particularly <40 mg/dl), high triglycerides (>150 mg/dl), and/or small LDL and increased VLDL, even if you don't have diabetes or pre-diabetes, selecting foods carefully based on glycemic index is very important. These patterns identify you as being at high genetic risk for diabetes. You should weigh your diet more heavily in favor of lean proteins like baked fish, baked (skinless) chicken and white meat turkey, egg whites, and low-fat dairy products such as cottage cheese and yogurt. You should choose non-starchy vegetables (all vegetables excluding white or sweet potatoes and corn) and non-starchy fruits (all fruits excluding bananas). Even if your blood sugar is normal, abnormally high blood sugar responses after meals are very common. Better control of blood sugar usually leads to an improvement in lipoprotein patterns. You should also consider a more comprehensive program to improve your "insulin sensitivity" (see box). Try to limit yourself to absolutely *no more than* two servings of starchy foods per day: bananas, whole grain breads, cereals, and other grain products. The bulk of your diet should be comprised of lean protein sources and non-starchy vegetables. Of course, all foods should be unrefined and whole whenever possible. When you do choose to indulge in a starchy food like a banana, try to combine it with sugar absorption slowing foods like raw nuts, sunflower seeds, pumpkin seeds, or oat bran. For example, you could combine a low-fat, unsweetened yogurt with sliced banana, but add sunflower seeds, oat bran, and strawberries.

Special considerations for diabetes and the metabolic syndrome

If you've already been diagnosed with diabetes (so-called type II only, or adult-onset; this discussion does not refer to type I, or juvenile, diabetes), borderline diabetes, or metabolic syndrome, all of the above principles apply to you, but even more so. In other words, these principles will, if applied appropriately, help you lose weight, lower blood sugar, and help correct lipoprotein disorders commonly associated with diabetes. However, you've likely been prescribed a diabetic diet by your doctor that limits your intake of carbohydrates and may encourage use of monounsaturated fats. (If you have not, you should request a formal consultation with a dietitian to discuss the details. This can be an important factor in your sugar control.) You should continue to adhere to this advice. **Track Your Plaque** principles should not interfere with a carbohydrate restriction nor with use of more monounsaturates. To compensate for the restriction in carbohydrates, you will have to increase your protein intake to accommodate the reduction in carbohydrate calories. You should therefore add more lean protein foods like baked fish, baked (skinless) chicken and white meat turkey, egg whites, and low-fat dairy products such as cottage cheese and yogurt. (If you have a history of kidney disease, or diabetic nephropathy, from your diabetes, you will need to discuss the advisability of increased protein intake with your doctor. Some nephrologists advocate a protein restriction when kidney disease develops.) Please be aware that following these guidelines can lead to significant drops in blood sugar. If you check your own sugars, you should continue to do so and inform your doctor of any consistent drops in blood sugar values. If you do not check your own sugars, you should discuss your blood sugar management with your doctor before making major changes in your diet.

Glycemic indexes for some common foods

This list is not meant to be complete, just to give you a good idea of where to start. As you get accustomed to looking at foods with glycemic index in mind, you will quickly be able to predict what a specific food's index will be without looking it up.

Whole, fiber-rich foods are nearly always low glycemic index, the best example of which are vegetables. The majority of foods in the undesirable high glycemic index list are carbohydrates. The difference in sugar responses between the highest and lowest glycemic index is *five-fold* (500%)! Note that, although whole wheat bread has fiber and other nutrients, its glycemic index is really not very different from white flour bread. It is still preferred over white bread for its superior nutrient content, but it provides no advantage from a glycemic index standpoint. Whole grain breads (usually made with oats) are somewhat better and are therefore found in the moderate glycemic index list.

You don't necessarily have to totally eliminate high glycemic index foods. Just minimize them. Use smaller portions and combine them with generous quantities of low glycemic index foods.

High glycemic index—Foods that raise blood sugar rapidly. These are mainly carbohydrates made of sugar and flour.
   Bananas
   Bread—white and whole wheat
   Candies
   Carrots
   Cereals—corn flakes, puffed rice, puffed wheat, Rice Krispies, granolas with
      added sugar, children's cereals
   Chips—potato, corn, taco
   Cookies

Corn
Donuts
Honey
Instant oatmeal
Pastries
Potatoes—white
Rice—white
Soft drinks and fruit drinks
Sugar

Moderate glycemic index
Applesauce
Barley
Beans—kidney, lima, pinto, black, red
Grapes
Multi-grain bread
Pasta—white or whole wheat
Peas
Oatmeal (non-instant)
Oranges, orange juice
Raisins
Yams, sweet potatoes

Low glycemic index—Cause blood sugar to rise slowly. These are often rich in fiber and most are non-carbohydrates or unprocessed foods. Please note that most whole fruits have a low glycemic index, but juices made from these fruits tend to have a high glycemic index, since much of the complex fibers have been removed.
Dairy products—milk, cottage cheese, ricotta cheese, yogurt (if unsweetened), cheeses
Egg whites, Egg Beaters
Fruit—Apples, pears, plums, peaches, grapefruit, cherries
Meats—chicken, fish, beef, pork
Nuts
Soybeans and soy products
Tomatoes, tomato sauce
Vegetables (non-starchy)—lettuce, green peppers, celery, broccoli, radishes, eggplant, cabbage, etc.

Principle No. 5: Create new habits

With so many different issues to consider, some people are overwhelmed when adopting these guidelines. You *will* need to break old habits. You'll likely find that, after learning the basic principles, you'll develop new healthy habits. Read labels and find foods that you enjoy. It's only an effort at first. Once you've established new habits, it becomes effortless.

Have you ever noticed how often you eat the same foods? For most of us, 10–20 different foods occupy 90% of the meals we eat over the course of a week. We then repeat these same 10–20 foods week after week. We may modify the preparation and mix combinations, but tend to rely on a relatively small number of foods. Following these guidelines really means just selecting a handful of healthy new foods and reorganizing your meals using these new choices. Many people get the mistaken notion that you will need to develop hundreds or thousands of new gourmet recipes in order to enjoy your new diet program. It's simply not true. Choose 10–20 basic dishes you enjoy and this will provide a basis for your broader diet. In fact, situations that offer unlimited variety, as in breakfast buffets or brunches, are where willpower crumbles. Stick to your healthy choices and avoid situations that tempt you to stray.

Here's a list of additional guidelines to help develop beneficial new habits:

- Eat vegetables, vegetables, and more vegetables. Occasionally add more vegetables. I'm exaggerating, but the point is to focus on vegetables over and above all other food sources. Vegetables are wonderfully versatile. Take advantage of the vast variety of vegetables as the basis of your nutrition program. Virtually all plant-based food sources are beneficial. Among the few exceptions are white potatoes and corn (high glycemic index). Vegetables are rich in fiber, have a low glycemic index, and are filling.

- Plant based foods in general, i.e., vegetables and fruits, beans, squash, etc., should be the *center of every meal* whenever possible, rather than meat. This way, side-dishes, even if not ideal foods, occupy less of your overall intake. For instance, make the main portion of your meal a vegetarian chili made with tomato sauce, beans, and other vegetables, along with a salad. On the side you might have a low-fat cheese burrito. While the burrito may have some saturated fat and refined flour, it occupies less of your overall meal.

- Always eat vegetables *first* and eat them in unlimited quantities. Seconds, thirds—as long as they're healthy vegetables, eat them in unrestricted quantities and fill up on them before you get to anything else. If there's any food that can be considered perfect, it's vegetables, and choosing them first will leave less room to indulge in other foods.

- Treat breads and other flour based products as *desserts*, rather than staples. Eat them sparingly and only after you've eaten more healthy foods like vegetables and fruits and lean proteins.

- Substitute fish for other meats whenever possible (for the omega-3 fatty acid content).

- Use healthy toppings and condiments: mustard, ketchup, horseradish, salsa; not mayonnaise, cheese sauces, gravies, etc. If you use oil based condiments, try to find brands made with canola, flaxseed, or olive oils. Be aware that most low or non-fat salad dressings are filled with high fructose corn syrup and should be avoided. Olive or canola oil based salad dressings are preferable.

- Do most of your grocery shopping in the outer aisles of the store, where you'll find the produce and dairy products. In this way, you'll avoid the temptations of the processed, high glycemic index foods in the center aisles.

You might consider the National Cancer Institute's (NCI) approach that urges men to consume *nine* servings of vegetables and fruits per day, women *seven* servings per day. Even though the NCI's advice is intended to reduce cancer risk, their approach can do the same for heart disease risk. (A "serving" means a cup of salad, a single whole fruit like one apple, or a half-cup of cut or chopped vegetables. A lunch that includes two cups of green salad and an orange, for example, would equal three servings.) Less than 10% of Americans currently eat this many fruits and vegetables.

If you're just starting to redesign your diet, you may spend a lot of time reading labels and experimenting with new foods and methods of preparation. Commit yourself to a few months of effort and you'll find that eating healthy will become second-nature.

Principle No. 6: Food should be enjoyed

At this point, perhaps some of you are saying, "How can I possibly enjoy eating if I'm unable to have so many of the foods I love?" At one time, I also shared this view. About 10 years ago, I visited the Pritikin Center in Miami Beach, Florida. Although their program differs from some of the principles of **Track Your Plaque** (there are many common aspects, as well), I learned that one great dietary success that the Pritikin Center accomplished was to elevate healthy eating to a gourmet level. The food was absolutely fabulous: tasty, beautifully presented, and fun. It was a convincing demonstration of just how interesting a healthy diet could be.

Until this experience, I had looked at dietary changes as a necessary sacrifice, leaving mostly bland and coarse foods. But this is simply untrue. A healthy diet can be every bit as interesting as an unhealthy one. In fact, my experience and that of many of my patients is that these changes usually lead to a *heightened* enjoyment of food. I think that people stop thinking about food as a momentary indulgence, and start regarding their diet as a creative activity that supports health. I frequently see patients rediscover delicious foods that had been lost in the pre-prepared, highly processed, fast food world they had previously lived in.

Making these changes is also best accomplished with a partner: your spouse, a close friend, your children. Psychological studies of the health habits of married couples clearly show that the eating and exercise practices of one partner very closely mirror that of the other. I've had occasional patients with a spouse who opposed changes in lifestyle. The spouse would refuse to quit smoking, or eliminate the Friday fish-fry or daily fast foods from their own habits and would not support changes for their partner. Success in this situation is difficult and rarely long lasting. The absence of support and ongoing temptations just erode your commitment. For this reason, I'll encourage the disinterested spouse to accompany the patient on office visits so that they're more likely to understand the rationale behind dramatic dietary changes. On several occasions, I've even had to advise marital counseling. The message: involve your partner. If they understand why you're making these changes in lifestyle, they're more inclined to support you. Whatever you need to do, such comprehensive changes in lifestyle are best accomplished as a shared experience.

It is human nature to stick to things we enjoy and find rewarding. We often end up rejecting things that we are forced to do. It is essential that you gravitate towards the foods and styles of preparation that make food enjoyable *for you*, rather than something you have to do for your health.

What about dietary vices—alcohol and caffeine?

Alcoholic drinks have their ups and downs. Obviously, if you have a drinking problem, no amount of alcohol is safe for you. The negative effects of excessive alcohol more than outweigh the modest benefits. On the positive side, alcoholic beverages can be part of the process of enjoying food. Many of my patients who've successfully followed **Track Your Plaque,** for instance, are wine enthusiasts. Evidence suggests that modest amounts of alcohol can lower heart attack risk. If you do choose to drink, deeply colored choices, especially red wines, are probably the most beneficial, as flavonoid content is greatest.

Moderation means only two glasses of wine per day for men, 1½ glasses for women (the lower amount for women due to body size). More than this and the adverse effects start to kick in: hypertension, increased triglycerides, and a net increase in heart attack risk. In addition, if you are overweight, alcohol can be a source of significant carbohydrate calories. This may be reason to minimize or eliminate alcoholic drinks while you are trying to lose weight.

Despite its ubiquity, caffeine has been a topic of controversy for many years. Several studies have suggested modest increases in blood pressure, but a clear cut association with heart disease is weak, at most. I suspect that there is indeed a barely measurable increase in heart disease risk with caffeine use and that the effect is dose dependent, i.e., the more you drink, the greater the adverse effect over a long period. Caffeine does, without argument, transiently raise blood pressure a small amount (generally 2–4 points). As high blood pressure is one of the potential ways to damage the lining of arteries, it is probably wise to limit your "dose" of caffeine to no more than approximately 250 mg per day: 2 cups of coffee, 3–4 cups of tea, 5–6 sodas (sugar free, of course).

Additional tips on creative healthy eating

You don't need to be a gourmet to enjoy creative food preparation. Like most of us, I look for foods that are healthy and delicious, but also not terribly difficult to prepare. Over the years, I've come across many simple strategies that can spice up your foods and make them interesting without sacrificing health. Some suggestions that may help you achieve success are:

- Experiment with spices: fresh or ground ginger, fresh basil, paprika, curry powder, nutmeg, and cilantro. Spices are a great way to avoid the use of salt, also. Peppers, hot sauces, sun-dried tomatoes, garlic, onion powder, curry powder—there are countless ways to make foods interesting without introducing artificial coloring or flavors.

- Switch to healthy condiments. Sample all the mustards available. There are a lot of choices: hot, yellow, brown, honey, horseradish, Dijon. They're fat free and versatile. If you haven't tried Wasabi sauce (Japanese horseradish), you'll be in for a treat. The taste is unique and it makes a great salad dressing or sauce. Ginger sauces, often with soy sauce, also make interesting accompaniments to fish and chicken. Balsamic vinegars are a whole world of their own and come in many varieties, ages, and regions of origin, much like wines. Likewise, wine vinegars and flavored vinegars can be used to vary your salad dressings. Hot pepper sauces can be a lot of fun on chicken or in vegetarian chili.

- Expand your vegetable choices. Try sun dried tomatoes, shiitaki mushrooms, various sprouts, and pea pods. Rediscover eggplant, radishes, squash, radicchio, raw spinach, and green onions. Deeply colored vegetables are tremendous sources of flavonoids, naturally occurring plant substances that lower cholesterol, lower blood pressure, and exert important non-cardiac effects, like reducing risk of cancer. Explore the world of alliums: scallions (green onions), red onions, white onions, Vidalia onions, shallots, leeks, chives, and garlic. They spice up your dishes whether raw or cooked, and are rich sources of phytonutrients and flavonoids.

- Add nuts and seeds (preferably raw) whenever possible. Walnuts, almonds, pecans, and sunflower seeds are easy additions to many dishes. They can add an interesting crunchy texture to salads (instead of flour based croutons). Raw nuts are rich in insoluble fiber, monounsaturated fats, phytonutrients, and even l-arginine. They can lower LDL cholesterol/particle number, lower Lp(a) to a modest degree, and slow digestion and increase the effective glycemic index of other foods. Dry roasted is okay only if not coated with sweeteners, not roasted in oil, etc., but raw is best.

- Use fruit to sweeten dishes. Try adding orange wedges, lemon or lime slices, apples, pears, strawberries, blueberries, apricots, etc. to salads and vegetable dishes for unexpected flavor and color combinations.

- Canned tomatoes are a convenient yet healthy time saver. They're great for adding to vegetable dishes or the basis for pasta sauces. Tomatoes are rich in phytonutrients, particularly lycopene, which has been shown to reduce LDL cholesterol and block its oxidation (to a more damaging form).

- Bits or slices of dried fruit make a great topping, e.g., on top of low-fat or non-fat cottage cheese or yogurt. Drying does serve to concentrate the sugar of the fruit, so be careful not to overdo it.

- When planning meals, vary the tastes of different dishes. You might try to include a selection with *sour* taste imparted by vinegars or lemons; *bitter* tastes from mustards, olives, and citrus rinds; *sweetness*, preferably from fruits, tomatoes, beets, yams and sweet potatoes, some squashes, beets, and honey (*not*, of course, from sugars, corn syrup, or high fructose corn syrup); and *hot* from peppers, garlic, and chili peppers. Interestingly, many people who crave fatty foods find satisfaction with hot foods, even without the expected steak, ground meat, etc. Try adding hot sauces and peppers to your healthy dishes if you are obliged to satisfy someone who insists on unhealthy foods.

- Make major meals, especially dinner, a joyful experience whenever possible. Plan a pleasant atmosphere: your patio, sunroom, outdoors, or with friends. Add candles or fresh flowers, turn on some background music (*not* the news). How could fast food ever replace this kind of intimate, sensual experience?

There you have it. Six basic principles and some useful tips to create a diet that you can use as a tool to control your coronary plaque. It is not a diet that will "cure" you of heart disease, but it is a program that helps ensure health from a variety of perspectives—lowers cancer risk, lowers blood pressure, helps control weight—and the foundation to your **Track Your Plaque** program. Let's review:

Summary: The six Track Your Plaque nutrition principles

Principle No. 1: Low-fat, good fat
Select foods rich in omega-3 and monounsaturated fatty acids; avoid saturated and hydrogenated fats as completely as possible.

Principle No. 2: Foods should be rich in fiber
Choose foods with knowledge of their soluble and insoluble fiber content and aim for an absolute minimum daily intake of 35 gm per day. High-fiber intakes help correct lipid/lipoprotein abnormalities, lower blood sugar and blood pressure, and help you lose weight.

Principle No.3: Foods should be unprocessed and unrefined
As often as possible, foods should be unprocessed—whole foods that are not extensively modified to enhance flavor and convenience. Unprocessed foods lack the glamour of processed, packaged foods, but are rich in fiber and nutrients, and lack additives that have adverse effects on lipoproteins.

Principle No. 4: Foods should have a low glycemic index
Weigh your diet more heavily towards foods that don't raise blood sugar dramatically. This helps turn-off the abnormal lipoprotein patterns that high blood sugar levels create, prevents diabetes, and avoids the hyperphagic (overeating) response that can lead to weight gain.

Principle No. 5: Create new habits
Redesign your habits by making new healthy choices and incorporate them into your life to make your new diet effortless.

Principle No. 6: Foods should be enjoyed

Make your initial sacrifices, but be certain to make food a fun, sensual experience that will keep you and your family interested.

In chapter 10, we discuss how to use exercise and the principle called "enhanced exercise" to help achieve your goal of correcting lipoprotein abnormalities and reducing your heart scan score.

Chapter 10

Control your plaque with exercise and weight-loss

Slash your need for medication and supercharge your program with these tips.

Step 3 of **Track Your Plaque** is to correct the lipid and lipoprotein abnormalities causing your coronary plaque. If you're eager to begin, exercise and weight-loss are tools you can start almost immediately* and add to specific lipoprotein treatments (chapter 8), nutritional strategies (chapter 9), and supplements (chapter 11).

I can almost always tell who does and who doesn't exercise when they walk into the office. The step of the exerciser is brisk and confident; they sit erect while we talk. Non-exercisers, in contrast, often drag their feet as they walk in and slump while they sit. The difference goes deeper than physical appearances. Exercisers are more upbeat and positive, less apt to stumble over the hurdles encountered in day-to-day life. They are more likely to deal effectively

---

* Before starting an exercise program, you should discuss the specifics of your program with your doctor first. Your doctor will be able to assess whether it is safe or not, given your particular starting condition. This is especially true if you have a positive heart scan score or a prior history of heart attack, angioplasty/stent, or bypass surgery, even if you are without symptoms. The actual risk of heart attack on initiating exercise when you start from a sedentary lifestyle is small, but it does happen. If your calcium score is >100, then a stress test prior to exercise is generally advisable, not to detect coronary disease, but to assess the safety of your response to exercise. This is true even if you don't have symptoms of chest pain, abnormal breathlessness, or neck or arm pain. If you do have any of these symptoms, a discussion with your doctor before undertaking exercise is an absolute necessity.

with change, both in their program, as well as life in general. To non-exercisers, hurdles in life often seem overwhelming, put there as obstacles to defeat them. When presented with change, they often resist and try to find an escape or excuse.

I've witnessed the transformation from a non-exerciser to an exerciser hundreds of times, but I am still amazed at the power in this process. Mike L. is a good example:

I met Mike at age 57. Two years earlier, Mike suffered a heart attack that converted the bottom third of his heart muscle to scar. His cardiologist at the time told him that the damage was done and the closed artery causing the heart attack could not be opened. They'd watch him for signs of an impending second heart attack. Mike accepted this answer but was dissatisfied with the lack of direction he was given in dealing with the causes of his heart disease.

When he came to me for a second opinion, Mike didn't walk, but lumbered slowly into the office. He plopped his 303 lbs. into a chair and slumped against the wall, huffing from the modest effort of walking 25 feet down the hallway, clearly not a physically active guy. Mike and I talked at length about how he needed to change his lifestyle, eating habits, correct his lipoprotein patterns (of which he had many), etc. I wasn't initially very hopeful that Mike could succeed in sacrificing his sedentary lifestyle dominated by snack filled TV watching.

To my surprise, Mike enthusiastically seized the exercise advice and launched a vigorous program of treadmill walking, the elliptical machine (a cross between a stair stepper and stationary bicycle), and weight training with light weights and high repetitions. He varied his routine but managed 45–60 minutes five days a week. Over a period of months, I saw Mike three more times. The transformation on each visit was impressive. By the end of six months, Mike had lost 60 lbs. He strode confidently into the office. He'd sit upright, eager to talk about his health. He'd learned to love exercise, as he experienced the power it had to change his health, mood, and appearance. For Mike, exercise provided a powerful tool for this tired, lethargic, and overweight man to regain control of his life.

The combination of exercise and weight-loss also yielded substantial improvement in Mike's lipoprotein abnormalities. Of course, he still required supplements and prescribed medicines to correct his lipid/lipoprotein patterns—he did suffer a heart attack, after all—but he viewed this as small price to pay for continued vigorous health.

Exercise can be a great self-empowering strategy for your program, something you can control. You can do a little or you can do a lot; it's up to you. It's also a natural method that costs little and can be fun. Likewise, weight-loss can achieve many of the same benefits. Combine the two, and you have a synergistic combination that yields substantial control over your heart disease future.

Participants in the program who exercise and maintain near ideal weight do enjoy greater success in controlling their heart scan score.

The discussion of how to exercise could fill an entire book by itself. There are many wonderful books, videos, and exercise programs that much more completely discuss the nuts and bolts of how to exercise. We will not cover these issues here. Our discussion will center around how exercise fits into the **Track Your Plaque** program to achieve improvements in lipid/lipoprotein patterns and gain control of your coronary plaque. Our discussion of weight-loss, similarly, will focus on how it can be used to advantage in the context of **Track Your Plaque** strategies. We will also discuss helpful strategies to accelerate the often frustrating weight-loss process.

"If I exercise hard enough, I'll never have a heart attack!"

Don't get the wrong idea: exercise is a means of minimizing, *not eliminating,* your need for other strategies. Men, in particular, are frequently guilty of this misguided attitude. They convince themselves that heart disease risk can be completely overpowered by vigorous exercise. Remember Tom from chapter 1? He was the marathon running, long distance biking architect with a high heart scan score. You may recall that Tom feared retracing his father's footsteps, so he committed himself to an extraordinarily rigorous exercise program to rid himself of heart disease risk. Exercise, even to Tom's extreme level, served to slow but not eliminate the growth of his coronary plaque. Unfortunately, exercise alone will not lower your heart scan score, nor will it completely turn-off your heart attack risk.

"If I eat right and take my medicines, do I really have to exercise?"

Conversely, can you succeed in shrinking your plaque yet be a complete couch potato? Perhaps. The price you'll pay will be more medication, a stricter diet, and an all around greater effort to achieve the same results. Inactive people really do struggle to succeed in controlling their health and are less likely to turn-off an increasing heart scan score. When I say "active", I don't mean like Tom. We'll discuss exactly what level of physical activity is required later in this section. For the most part, the level of physical activity required to succeed is modest, a level that just about anybody can reach. Luck eventually runs out for the couch potato if sedentary habits lead to substantial weight gain, as it nearly always does. Once inactivity leads to obesity, it commonly leads to glucose intolerance (pre-diabetes, or metabolic syndrome) and diabetes, and control of your score becomes extremely difficult. Even if obesity isn't yet present, inactivity all by itself can still result in insulin resistance (a prerequisite for developing diabetes) and all its associated lipoprotein disturbances.

"But I don't want to be an athlete!"

Let's distinguish two different goals in an exercise program. The goal for **Track Your Plaque** purposes is to use exercise to help reduce risk of heart attack and shrink coronary plaque. This requires a level of physical activity that just about anyone can reach with a modest commitment of time and effort. A very different goal is to achieve a high level of cardiovascular fitness like a competitive athlete. This distinction may seem obvious. Many people, when a modest exercise program is suggested to reduce cardiovascular risk, instead hear "I want you to achieve extreme levels of cardiovascular fitness!" They are intimidated, fearing hours upon hours of exercising to exhaustion, and give up before they've even started. Extreme fitness is simply not necessary to obtain significant cardiovascular benefits.

The truth is that almost anybody can reach the levels of physical effort required to achieve your goals in **Track Your Plaque.** The people at The Cooper Aerobics Center in Dallas, Texas have accumulated a vast experience in observing how physical fitness impacts on heart attack risk. All participants in the Cooper programs undergo stress testing as a measure of fitness when they enroll. Their studies show that the bulk of protective benefit of exercise come from walking, light yard work, and other similar but modest levels of everyday activities. Surprisingly, higher levels of fitness—long distance jogging, long distance biking, etc.—provide only a slight additional decrease in heart attack risk.

The broad health enhancing benefits of exercise are undisputed. Let's now talk more specifically about how exercise and weight control can be used as tools to keep your heart scan score from increasing. We achieve this, once again, by using exercise to help correct your lipid and lipoprotein patterns.

Exercise—a treatment for lipids and lipoproteins

What are the beneficial lipid and lipoprotein effects of exercise? Let's list them:

- Exercise *increases HDL cholesterol.* Going from a sedentary couch potato to moderate activity, most people raise HDL by around five points. This effect lasts about two weeks. The majority of people can achieve this level of benefit without expending extraordinary effort. Extreme levels of exercise can raise HDL 10 points if sustained. Exercise increases the most beneficial HDL2 fraction, or large, HDL more than the less beneficial HDL3, or small, HDL.

- Exercise *decreases triglycerides.* This effect can be significant, particularly if exercise leads to weight-loss. Drops of 100 points are not uncommon if exercise is sustained and consistent.
- Exercise *decreases LDL cholesterol and LDL particle number/apoprotein B.* This is a modest effect. Reductions in LDL of 10% are common—enough to help when part of a more comprehensive effort, though usually not enough to stand alone.
- Exercise *increases LDL particle size.* This effect goes hand in hand with the rise in HDL cholesterol. Exercise by itself will rarely fully correct this pattern but can be a useful adjunct to other therapies.
- Exercise *lowers blood pressure.* Exercise generally yields a drop of two to four points when sustained and consistent.
- Exercise *lowers blood sugar.* Many people with borderline diabetic tendencies can improve sensitivity to their body's insulin by consistent physical activity.
- Exercise *helps control weight.* Weight-loss magnifies all of the above listed lipoprotein benefits and lowers blood sugar, as well. Exercise makes weight-loss efforts more successful by contributing to the 3500 calories required to lose a pound of weight. Even if you're already at your desired weight, exercise makes maintaining weight much easier.

Exercise also makes you feel better. Once you make exercise a consistent activity several times a week, you will likely experience improved mood, deeper sleep, greater alertness, clearer and more optimistic thinking. People who are brighter in their overall outlook tend to be more successful in other spheres of life. They are also less likely to indulge in mood elevating but health defeating habits like smoking, excessive drinking, and too much caffeine. All this can translate into greater success in correcting lipoprotein abnormalities.

Unfortunately, not all abnormalities are improved by exercise. Lp(a) and homocysteine are the most resistant, remaining virtually unchanged even if you attain elite levels of athletic training. For correction of these abnormalities, refer to the treatments discussed in chapter 8.

The benefits of exercise are not permanent. Even if you were an Olympic level athlete in high school or college, the benefits of training dissipate over a period of months after you stop. It's not so much *what* you do, as how long and consistently you do it. Modest efforts carried out over a period of 10 years yield far greater benefits than intensive exercise for six months followed by sporadic efforts. Some of the most successful participants in **Track Your Plaque** are people who've committed themselves to very modest, yet realistic, exercise routines, such as walking with a spouse for 30 minutes, four times a week. This is not physically challenging for most people, but does require a commitment to follow through, with consistent effort week after week, month after month, year after year.

The secret to a successful exercise program

Take a practical, long-term perspective and answer the following question: "What sorts of physical activities can I perform and stick to for the next 30 years—and enjoy doing it?" The key here is not the form or intensity of effort. *The essential ingredient is that you derive some form of enjoyment from the activity.* If you force yourself to pedal five miles a day on a stationary bicycle in your basement but despise every moment of it, you're unlikely to succeed over the long-haul. People who discover enjoyment and satisfaction in their exercise will stick to their program, even when stressful distractions crop up in other parts of their lives.

For some people, solitary activities that provide quiet moments for contemplation might be desirable, such as walking on a treadmill, riding a bicycle, or using an elliptical machine. Others prefer the camaraderie and sense of shared experience that is only possible in larger groups. For these people, aerobic classes, group yoga instruction, spinning classes and other organized group activities might be best. Still others might most enjoy the close company of a partner on walks, tennis, golf, etc.

Perhaps you need to be mentally stimulated—you're bored easily and struggle to exercise more than a few minutes. If you prefer visual stimulation, you might do better by watching the news on TV while on your stationary bike. If you prefer auditory stimulation, listen to some of your favorite CD's or the radio while you walk a treadmill. You might vary your choice of exercise over the course of a week: bike once a week, walk twice a week, swim once a week, play tennis once a week. The point is to succeed by enjoying yourself. Do things you like and you might even look forward to it.

What happened to "No pain, no gain?"

What constitutes a sufficient level of physical activity? For instance, is light to moderate gardening good enough? How about cutting grass? Do you have to exercise to exhaustion or is just breaking a light sweat enough?

You can decide for yourself whether an activity is sufficiently stimulating to the cardiovascular system if you raise and sustain your heart rate to *70% of your age-predicted maximum heart rate or greater.* This seems like an awfully complex rule, but it's really simple to calculate. To get your 70% target (the minimum heart rate you would like to achieve and sustain), start with the number 220 and subtract your age; multiply the result by 0.7 (70%). This will give you the approximate *minimum* heart rate required to yield the sorts of benefits listed earlier. (This applies to both men and women.) For example, if you're 50 years old:

$$220-50 = 170$$
$$170 \times 0.7 = 119$$

You therefore need to maintain your heart rate at 119 beats per minute or greater. A heart rate of 119 is easy to attain by a brisk walk, light to moderate effort biking, walking on your treadmill with a modest incline (say, 3% grade), raking leaves, singles tennis, and ballroom dancing, just to name a few examples. Measure your heart rate by feeling the pulse in your wrist (just below the base of your thumb). Count the number of heart beats in 15 seconds and multiply times four; this yields heart beats per minute. You can also measure your heart rate by using one of the many heart rate monitors available today or that come built into exercise machines. These devices are reasonably accurate. If you have cause to doubt a device's accuracy, just compare the heart rate readout to the value you obtain by taking your pulse. You can, of course, exceed this 70% level (provided your doctor agrees). You will burn more calories and lose more weight, but the additional improvement in your lipids and lipoproteins will be relatively small.

The "no pain, no gain" mantra does not apply to you. This is meant for people whose aim is to achieve higher levels of fitness for competition, or other such purposes that have little to do with our goals. Pain is not required to achieve success in correcting lipids/lipoproteins or losing weight. Much of the benefit from exercise comes by devoting sufficient *time* to your efforts. Two hours a week of a 70% effort is the minimum, preferably divided up into three or four sessions. This amount provides 90% of the lipid/lipoprotein benefits achievable with exercise. Less than this and you might not obtain the improvements in lipoprotein patterns you desire. More than this, and there are modest additional increments of only 10% in your lipoproteins. (This does not mean that lipoprotein abnormalities are 100% correctable with exercise. It simply means that vigorous exercise can improve lipids/lipoproteins, and exercising at the level described above will achieve 90% of this amount.) The message is that intense exercise is not necessary for you to feel better, lose weight, or correct your lipids and lipoproteins.

Lose weight faster with exercise

The closer you are to your ideal weight, the more likely you'll succeed in controlling the growth of plaque in your coronary arteries. If you are significantly overweight, success is still possible but other efforts (exercise, diet, medical treatments, etc.) will be correspondingly greater. Excess fat (particularly when concentrated in the abdomen) produces several evil substances known as "adipocytokines". These molecules appear to be responsible for many of the negative effects of excess weight, particularly high blood levels of fatty acids and resistance to insulin. (Research in this same area yielded the recent discovery of leptin, a hormone that may be responsible for appetite control. This will be an exciting area of investigation in the coming years.)

Some lipoprotein patterns are very sensitive to body weight. If you begin with a low HDL, high triglycerides and VLDL, or small LDL particles, all of these abnormalities improve with weight-loss. (If you have these abnormalities but are not overweight, then no further benefit will be obtained by losing weight.) The number of pounds required to correct each pattern differs widely from person to person. In general, however, the effect can be significant. Increases in HDL of 5–10 points and decreases of >50 in triglycerides are common when losing 10–20 pounds, for instance.

Losing weight is almost always best accomplished with a combi-

---

Am I overweight?

Let's face it: most of us know when we are overweight. But if you need a measure to establish a baseline and track to assess your results, one helpful number is the Body Mass Index, or BMI. Many studies examining the health risks of excess weight use the BMI.

BMI is calculated using your height and weight. What it does not take into account is your relative bone structure ("I'm big-boned") or the relative proportion of muscle mass compared to fat that you have. Different races can also have distorting effects on the BMI. In other words, the BMI is a rough index that tends to lump many different body types together based purely on size.

To calculate your BMI:

1) Weight in kilograms (kg) = weight in pounds ÷ 2.2

2) Height in meters (m) = height in inches x 0.025

3) BMI = weight (kg) ̷ height (m) 2

A BMI of 20-25 is ideal, 25-30 is overweight, and >30 is obese.

Another helpful measure that eliminates the differences in body types is *body fat percent*, most readily obtained with bioimpedance devices (body fat analyzers), now inexpensive and widely available in health clubs and stores (discussed in more detail later in this chapter). If your percent body fat exceeds 25% for males or 33% for females, then you are overweight, and this likely contributes to your lipoprotein abnormalities. Percent body fat can provide great feedback to track your results as you proceed through exercise and weight-loss efforts.

---

nation of diet and exercise. It is very difficult to lose any more than a few pounds relying exclusively on diet only, while neglecting exercise, or vice versa. Remember that losing one pound means you need to burn 3500 calories more than you consume in food. Achieving this with calorie restriction alone is tough. Few people successfully lose weight and keep it off using diet alone. This principle was demonstrated very clearly by Mike and Darlene:

Remember Mike's transformation from an overweight, lethargic, survivor of a heart attack to the vigorous, energetic exercise enthusiast?

Mike, 57, and his wife, Darlene, 58, were both significantly overweight when I first met them. At the start, Mike, at 6 feet 2 inches, was 303 lbs. Darlene, at 5 feet 1 inch, was 203 lbs. Both had multiple lipoprotein abnormalities that could improve markedly with weight-loss and exercise, including low HDL, small LDL, excess VLDL and triglycerides. In addition, Mike was borderline diabetic and had already been started on a diabetic medication by his family doctor. This close couple, married 23 years, had committed to better health together and wished to proceed through the program as partners. The couple was interested in minimizing the use of medication to correct their lipoprotein disorders and so jumped wholeheartedly into a nutrition program (like the one described in chapter 9) and exercise. The couple exercised for 45–60 minutes (actually more than the recommended time) five days a week, Darlene by walking, biking, and aerobics; Mike by a combination of walking a treadmill, elliptical trainer, and weight training. After six months, Mike had lost 60 lbs; Darlene lost 50 lbs—phenomenal results. The couple was ecstatic and would walk into my office beaming with pride over their success.

Unfortunately, family stresses entered their lives that took the greatest toll on Darlene. Their 29-year-old daughter with three young children was going through a messy divorce. Darlene had no choice but to devote much of her time and emotional energy to helping her daughter deal with this life shattering change, and Darlene sacrificed her exercise efforts in the process. At the same time, Mike did try to do his part but still managed to maintain his exercise routine. Another six months later, Mike was looking great, having maintained his ideal weight and avoided regaining the 60 lbs. he'd lost. Darlene, on the other hand, because of the unselfish devotion to her daughter's children, regained the entire 50 lbs over the next year, even though she'd been meticulous in adhering to her diet. She felt overwhelmed and defeated.

The lesson: despite good nutritional habits followed by both, it was the *exercise* that allowed Mike to maintain his weight, while Darlene's (understandable) lapse in exercise led her right back to her original overweight condition. Darlene's experience is somewhat extreme but nonetheless an example of how the combined effects of exercise and diet yielded the greatest results.

The key in using exercise to burn off calories and lose weight is more the *duration* of exercise, and not the intensity. For instance, a relaxed 40-minute walk on your treadmill at 3.2 miles per hour and 3% incline, while maintaining a heart rate of 120, will get you better results than a hard walk for 20 minutes. Losing weight will require you to exercise longer than if you were just trying to maintain weight. Exercising 30 minutes per session is best for maintaining weight; *longer* periods are required to burn the additional calories to achieve weight-loss.

Muscle burns calories

If you're trying to lose weight, consider weight or strength training.

As we age, we lose muscle mass and gain fat. At age 65, the average man has lost 30% or more of his muscle mass, a woman at least 20%. Muscles are calorie furnaces and a youthful quantity of muscle can help burn fat. Greater muscle mass increases your body's basal metabolic consumption of calories. In other words, muscle consumes calories just to meet its energy requirements. This means you're burning up calories without trying, just from the heightened metabolic requirements of muscle. You don't have to be a bodybuilder to achieve these modest benefits, and neither will you bulge with muscles.

You can obtain significant calorie burning benefits of muscle just by weight training once or twice a week for 20 minutes per session—a very modest time investment. If you're unfamiliar with the machines or free weight movements, most health clubs can provide instruction to get you started. Once you're shown the basic movements, the rest is really quite easy. Follow a circuit-training approach using higher repetitions (10–20) at each station with little or no rest in between, and the 20 minutes you devote to weight training will also suffice as aerobic exercise. (Circuit-training refers to following a sequence of strength exercises in a cycle that you can repeat several times; ask your trainer specifically about this technique.)

If you incorporate weight training, you will add muscle weight (often several pounds) and your net weight-loss from fat may not seem as dramatic. If you choose to add weight or strength-training to your program, assessing just how much fat-weight reduction you've achieved is easy. There are two ways to do this:

1. Measure body fat percent. Convenient devices to measure body fat are widely available nowadays. Reliable units cost as little as $50. (Tanita manufactures several great products.) Many health spas and clubs now have them, as well. Body fat is measured using bio-impedance, which makes use of the differing electrical conductivity of fat and muscle. (Muscle is a conductor of electricity; fat is an insulator.) A very small quantity of electrical current (which you cannot feel) is passed through the body and the device calculates how much fat and muscle is encountered in the path of the current. Devices that pass the current through the feet ("foot-to-foot"), as opposed to the hands ("hand-to-hand"), are more reliable. You

stand on these devices much like a conventional scale. Current passed from one hand to the other is a better measure of fat and muscle in the thorax, but neglects much of the abdomen. Foot-to-foot bio-impedance includes the abdomen and tends to be more accurate, particularly if you have excess abdominal fat characteristic of the metabolic syndrome. Body fat can also be measured by using calipers and measuring the thickness of fat in several skin folds around the body. This is best performed by someone who does this frequently, such as a personal trainer. If you do it yourself, there is just too much room for "fudging" results.

2. Look in the mirror. This may sound obvious but it can really provide useful feedback If you gain muscle and lose fat, you'll notice a more erect posture; broader shoulders; a flatter, more muscular abdomen, firmer thighs. After all, most people are very interested in looking good and weight training can really yield great improvements in appearance.

"I'm not losing weight fast enough!"

With two pregnancies, the pressures of raising children, a near full-time job in real estate sales, and neglect of her own health, Jan had gained 75 lbs. At age 47, Jan now tipped the scales at 193 lbs., her heaviest ever. She'd tried several diets over the years as well as exercise, though inconsistently, with limited success. But the long-term trend was dismayingly upward.

Jan's excess weight eventually made her wonder if she was at risk for heart disease, since both parents succumbed in their 60's. Jan underwent a heart scan. Her score: 154 (>90th percentile). Lipoprotein testing revealed six abnormalities that would improve substantially with weight reduction (low total and large HDL, elevated triglycerides and VLDL, small LDL, and increased LDL particle number). As Jan preferred healthy approaches to medication, she expressed great interest in learning how to successfully lose weight. She declared to me, "I want to lose 40 lbs in the next two months!"

Jan is a typical example. Once they find out that they have hidden heart disease and that excess weight is like gasoline on the fire of coronary plaque, people are suddenly motivated to lose weight quickly. Despite the fact that it required decades to gain the weight, most want *immediate* results, not complicated formulas, long exercise routines, etc. Unfortunately, there's no safe method that results in meaningful weight-loss without effort, but there are several methods that can *accelerate* weight-loss to a modest degree and get your weight to goal faster.

Let's first dispense with so-called "thermogenic" agents, potentially hazardous substances that increase the body's metabolic rate. They increase heart rate and blood pressure and essentially act as a gas pedal for your body's fat burning rate. These agents include ephedra, ma huang, guarana, bitter orange, and pseude-phedrine. One or more of these agents is often "stacked" with aspirin and caffeine to compound the metabolism accelerating effect. Thermogenic agents are mod-erately effective for weight-loss, but they can also be dangerous. The FDA has already banned the sale of phenylpropanolamine and ephedra because of their association with stroke and heart attack. You are strongly advised not to use these preparations singly or in combination. The risks are simply not worth it, particu-larly if you have coronary plaque.

Calcium pyruvate

Calcium pyruvate is one of the few effective nutritional supplements for weight-loss. Though it helps accelerate fat burning, it is not a thermogenic agent and shares none of their dangerous effects. At one time, calcium pyru-vate was slated to be a prescription weight-loss agent, but instead was released as a nutritional supplement. The exact mechanism for calcium pyruvate's weight-loss accelerating effect is not clear, but likely relates to enhanced energy production in the body, as pyruvate is a participant in ATP synthesis (the mol-ecule that provides the body's energy). The dose that works best is 2.5 grams (2500 milligrams) twice a day. If you were destined to lose five pounds on your diet without calcium pyrvuate, you might lose seven pounds instead by taking 2.5 grams twice a day—not a huge effect, but still helpful.

Calcium pyruvate works best, however, as an "exercise enhancer". Take 2.5 grams one hour before exercise and most people feel like they can exercise longer and harder. Exercising is more pleasant and you also won't be as sore the next day. Used in this fashion, many people lose weight more rapidly and have more fun in the process, since exercise is just a more pleasant experience. You can use calcium pyruvate strictly as an "exercise enhancer" at 2.5 grams prior to your work-out, or you can take 2.5 grams twice a day with one of the doses one hour before exercise. The second regimen is slightly more effective in shedding weight.

Calcium pyruvate has few side-effects beyond mild nausea, and even this is rare. For unclear reasons, calcium pyruvate doesn't work for everybody and the only way to find out is to give it a try.

Several other supplements or agents that are worth mentioning that can be helpful in selected individuals are:

Progesterone

Progesterone is a fascinating weight-loss accelerating tool for women that may even provide youth preserving benefits, as well.

Progesterone is useful only to females age 35 and over as the peri-menopausal phase of life begins to get underway, and for women who are menopausal. Don't confuse progesterone with estrogen, which has an entirely different panel of good and bad effects. As a woman proceeds through the peri-menopause, she often notices that weight becomes harder to control, even if she makes no change in diet or exercise. Some of this effect is attributable to diminishing levels of progesterone in the body. Many women also experience fatigue, sleeplessness or inability to sleep deeply, lack of physical energy, and feelings of hopelessness or sadness. After menopause, *all* women are deficient in progesterone compared to pre-menopausal women. Many of the effects of low progesterone improve with progesterone replacement. Commonly, when a woman begins progesterone (e.g., cream preparations that you can rub on the chest and arms), within four to eight weeks she gains physical energy, sleeps more deeply, experiences a gradual improvement in mood, and losing weight gets easier—sort of like turning the clock back 10 years. For these reasons, progesterone is a very popular ingredient among the anti-aging community.

Having prescribed progesterone cream to many of my female patients, I can attest to its beneficial effects. The only side-effect is the expected resumption of menses in menopausal women on the days when progesterone is not taken. (Most women, unless they've had a hysterectomy, apply progesterone cream 25 days out of 30, with light vaginal bleeding on the five days without progesterone.) Weight-loss is modest and gradual and still dependent on diet and exercise efforts. In other words, you will not immediately shed pounds just by adding progesterone. But you may find that less effort is required to lose weight. Doses of 25 mg twice a day for women before menopause, 50 mg twice a day during and after menopause have worked well. Doses can also be adjusted by your doctor, depending on your response. Natural progesterone creams can be prepared to your doctor's specifications through special pharmacies called "compounding" pharmacies. (Compounding pharmacies are usually listed as such in the yellow pages. Also, see Appendix D.)

The issue of progesterone is complex and never fails to stimulate controversy. More and more gynecologists are adopting the use of natural progesterone creams (available both by prescription and over-the-counter), though a great many still remain ignorant of its benefits. A discussion of this fascinating hormone could easily fill an entire book. If the idea of progesterone replacement interests you, I would urge you to read further. The most concise summary of the history and use of progesterone can be found in Dr. John Lee's books, *What Your Doctor May Not Tell You About Pre-Menopause* and *What Your Doctor May Not Tell You About Menopause* (Warner Books).

Testosterone

Analogous to a woman's progesterone, levels of testosterone in the male diminish after age 30, leading to progressive loss of muscle mass, increased body fat, declining libido, low moods and even depression. These changes are most dramatic after a man passes beyond his mid-40s. Some call this time the "male menopause," or "andropause." Since there is no visible change in a man's life like the cessation of menstruation in a woman, the onset of this phase of life can be very subtle and usually dismissed as "getting old."

Nonetheless, testosterone replacement can be one helpful way for men to feel more vigorous, gain muscle strength, partially restore lost libido, as well as help control weight. As with progesterone, testosterone replacement does not result in a prompt drop in weight, but simply makes losing a few pounds easier, similar to the ease experienced when you were younger.

Testosterone is also a controversial treatment that is fraught with unfounded fears and misperceptions. It does not, for instance, convert normal men into "sex maniacs." It may restore a more youthful sex drive, often similar to that experienced in your 30's. Men who feel run down, lack energy, and wish to accelerate weight-loss might consider testosterone cream, one method of replacement. This requires a prescription and can be formulated for you by special pharmacies (compounding pharmacies). Testosterone can also be obtained as prescription patches, gel patches, or injections. (The prescribed dose depends on the form used and your response.) Avoid oral testosterone, as this is associated with serious liver side-effects. You may find that many doctors will shy away from prescribing testosterone to enhance your mood, energy, etc, and prefer to prescribe it only for a condition called hypogonadism, which is a severe, abnormal lack of testosterone. A frank, open discussion with your doctor to discuss your interests may help persuade him/her to prescribe testosterone. In my practice, I prescribe testosterone to men over age 40 if the above symptoms are present and total testosterone level is less than 450, or if the free (non-protein bound) testosterone is low (in the lower half of the normal range for the laboratory used). Some concern has been raised that administration of testosterone may cause a hidden prostate cancer to grow, though this has not been documented in any clinical study. Nonetheless, it is probably wise to have both a prostate exam and a prostate specific antigen (PSA) test prior to starting testosterone and annually thereafter.

DHEA

DHEA (dihydroepiandrosterone) is a hormone produced in the adrenal glands that is a close "cousin" of estrogen and testosterone. Despite being amongst the most abundant of the body's hormones in both men and women, the function of DHEA is not well understood despite thousands of clinical studies examining its role in bodily functions. It is clear, however, that low DHEA levels are associated with lack of energy, depressed mood, loss of muscle and increased fat. DHEA levels diminish gradually as we age, such that the level in most people over 70 years old is nearly unmeasurable. DHEA replacement's most prominent benefits are improved mood and energy. In fact, DHEA has been used successfully for treatment of severe depression. It is especially effective for boosting the "blahs", feelings of lethargy and disinterest that plague many of us in our 40s and onwards. With sleep, DHEA's effects can be paradoxical and unpredictable. Some people experience deep, satisfying sleep when taking DHEA; others suffer insomnia. The reason for the varying response is not clear.

Does DHEA help you lose weight? The effect is subtle and may relate more to the increase in physical energy and mood, rather than a direct weight-loss effect. If, with DHEA replacement, you're more energetic and upbeat, you are also more likely to exercise, eat healthy foods, and not indulge in mood elevating behaviors like binge-feeding on sweets, smoking, and alcohol. The weight-loss effect may be most significant if you take your DHEA at bedtime (if you are among the lucky 50% who enjoy deep sleep rather than insomnia) because DHEA has been shown to increase effective growth hormone levels in the body by 30%. Growth hormone plays a crucial role in maintaining youthful characteristics, including weight control.

DHEA is best taken with the assistance of your physician, since your DHEA sulfate (DHEA-S) level should be checked prior to beginning DHEA replacement. The great majority of people 40 years old and over have levels of <400 ng/dl. If your level is higher than 400, you likely will not benefit much from DHEA supplementation. A repeat DHEA-S level should be checked four weeks after starting supplementation to avoid exceeding the upper limits of normal (specified by the laboratory where the test is run). DHEA supplementation should only be considered by people 40 years old and above, when the DHEA level in your body has likely dropped to half that of a 20 year old. A good starting dose is 25 mg and then adjusted to your level of DHEA-S. Rarely is more than 50 mg per day required to achieve the desired effects. Some people have expressed concerns about the unknown effects of artificially elevated DHEA levels in the body, including cancer, but none of these have ever materialized in any study. In my experience, DHEA has been safe and effective when used properly. In years past, people were guilty of using much higher doses of DHEA of up to 300 mg. This is when you see unwanted side-effects: aggressive behaviors, hirsutism (mustaches) in females, increased testosterone in females and increased estrogen in males. These effects are rarely seen at doses below 50 mg per day. DHEA is not advised if you are diabetic or if you are pre-diabetic, as DHEA will tip the scales in favor of more insulin resistance.

There are several other products that are popularly promoted to accelerate weight-loss. However, the existing scientific data and our experience with these agents have suggested no positive effects. These include hydroxycitric acid, conjugated linolenic acid, and l-carnitine. I would not recommend use of these supplements to accelerate weight-loss. (This hasn't stopped many promoters from making extravagant claims about these agents, however.)

Carbohydrate restriction—Nutritional strategy to super-charge weight-loss

There's no doubt about it. Carbohydrate restricted diets do yield greater weight-loss results. While skepticism slowed the acceptance of these diets, more recent clinical studies confirm that carbohydrate restriction does indeed result in greater immediate weight-loss than low-fat diets. The Atkins diet, South Beach Diet, the Zone diet, Sugar-busters, etc. all advocate somewhat similar diets that restrict carbohydrates—pasta, breads, potatoes, flour containing products, cakes, cookies, even fruits. These programs are higher in proteins and oils to make up for the reduced carbohydrates.

While following the **Track Your Plaque** nutrition principles can yield significant weight-loss, adding a carbohydrate restriction can amplify this effect. You might therefore choose to borrow some of the principles from one of these diets if weight-loss is a major interest for you.

Any of these diets are reasonable approaches to follow to augment your weight-loss efforts. They all advocate slashing carbohydrate calories from the usual highly-refined starch diet of most Americans. The Atkins approach allows indiscriminate intake of high saturated fat sources like cheese, bacon, and red meats in its induction phase. The others are somewhat more selective. The Zone, for instance, dictates specific proportions of calories from fats, proteins, and carbohydrates based on their effects on prostaglandins. Despite some differences in philosophy in the beginning stages, all these diets in their later phases gravitate towards a common program of balanced intakes of carbohydrates, fats, and protein that is not very different from a diet crafted from the **Track Your Plaque** nutrition principles.

Once your weight-loss efforts are attained, you should return to a diet *for health,* such as that detailed in chapter 9 of **Track Your Plaque.** The nutrition principles detailed in this book yield significant improvements in lipoproteins and thereby coronary plaque control, and are therefore part of a program for long-term health, not just weight-loss.

Interestingly, the people most likely to respond to a carbohydrate restricted diet are people with excessive carbohydrate sensitivity. You can recognize these people by their lower HDL's (<50 mg/dl), higher triglycerides (>150 mg/dl), small LDL, and body shape characterized by excess abdominal weight (metabolic syndrome). People with these common features tend to respond to carbohydrate restricted diets with a faster than usual drop in weight. The Atkins diet, in particular, advocates (in its induction phase) unlimited intake of saturated fat sources. This is safe if done for only a few weeks at a time and, contrary to popular fears, usually does not result in a rise in LDL (or LDL particle number or apoprotein B). This is probably due to the dramatic reduction in VLDL when carbohydrates are slashed from the diet, since VLDL yields LDL.

Caloric expenditure—Keeping you honest

Time after time, people say, "I don't understand it. I'm eating healthy foods and exercising, but I'm just not losing any weight!"

Measure the number of calories these people burn in physical activity during the course of a day, and they commonly fall far short of the average person's daily energy usage. In other words, many people have gotten overweight because they've become very economical in their physical activity. The next time you're at work or in public, observe how overweight people move. They will often be very spare in their motions. They'll be seated at a desk and scoot about in their wheeled desk chair, rather than get up. They will reach for things, rather than get up and walk to get it. They'll use more hand motion rather than their body and legs. Each one of these economies of movement may conserve only a fraction of a calorie, but compounded hour after hour, day after day, and it all adds up to a progressive gain in weight. These people are very efficient in their calorie burning, and the unburned energy is saved as fat. When you measure the amount of energy people burn, overweight people burn far less calories—often *half* or less the calorie expenditure compared to a non-overweight person.

You can measure your calorie expenditure using a very clever device called a pedometer. Pedometers have come a long way since the crude mechanical devices available when we were kids. I've used several excellent models that cost between $10–20. You can find them in sporting goods stores, health clubs, and in some department stores. Present day pedometers can measure horizontal motion fairly accurately and convert this to number of calories burned. You can, therefore, use a pedometer to measure how active you are and how many calories you're actually expending. Sedentary, overweight people who wear a pedometer commonly burn only 100–150 calories in a typical 12 hour day. (This is over and above the basal metabolic rate requirement.) Active people, on the other hand, commonly burn 350–500 or more calories. The daily difference is not great, perhaps 200 calories. But the 200 cal/day difference leads to a one lb. weight gain over 17.5 days (3500÷200 = 17.5). Over a year: 21 lbs.! That's 21 lbs. just from subconsciously limiting movement through an ordinary day.

Another common difficulty is that, when you cut your calorie intake, your body's survival instincts kick in and you unconsciously cut back on physical activity. Some call this resetting your "set-point". This instinctive behavior served humans well when we had to forage for food during times of starvation. A reduction in calorie intake triggers our bodies to conserve energy. We reduce energy expenditure, though in almost imperceptible ways. Like the people who gain weight because of more economical movements, you will also limit your energy expenditure by cutting corners in your daily physical activities. However, if you are aware of this subconscious phenomenon, you can use it to your advantage by consciously resisting the inertia to physical activity—get up and get going!

Before starting your weight-loss program, wear the pedometer and record the number of calories you burn each day over a specific period. For example, reset your pedometer starting at 8 a.m., then go through your day. At 8 pm, write down the total calories burned. This provides a good idea of how many calories you've expended through the most active part of your day. If you've used only 175 calories, you know that you've had a relatively inactive day. If you've used 350 calories, this has been a moderately active day that will help control weight. Repeat this process for three successive days and average the daily value.

Once you've determined the average number of calories you burn each day, you can now set your goals higher. A goal of 350 calories in a 12 hour period is realistic. If you fall short, you can review your day and see how you might do better the next day—avoid shortcuts when you're shopping, parking farther away at the office, walking an extra five minutes on your treadmill, etc. Increasing your energy expenditure (without increasing your calorie intake) by only 100 calories a day will result in a loss of one pound a month or 12 pounds a year—quite significant over a long period. (Certain activities, like swimming or biking, cannot be properly quantified by most pedometers.) If you are in a hurry to lose weight, you can increase your daily expenditure accordingly. For example, adding another 230 calories of calorie expenditure per day (it's really not that tough) will result in weight-loss of two pounds per month over and above what you achieve by other efforts.

Combine weight-loss tools for faster results

If you're in a hurry to lose weight to gain control of your lipid/lipoprotein abnormalities and coronary plaque, then combine weight-loss tools to super-charge your results.

For instance, use calcium pyruvate 2.5 gm twice a day with one dose prior to your exercise routine. Add an additional 10 minutes to your usual 25 minutes and increase your daily calorie expenditure (outside of exercise) to 450 calories per day using your pedometer. If agreeable to your doctor, add 25 mg DHEA at bedtime and progesterone or testosterone cream. Follow the **Track Your Plaque** nutrition principles but pay attention to slashing your carbohydrate intake and completely eliminate breads, pastas, dairy products, and fruits for four weeks.

This multi-pronged attack on weight is extremely effective and commonly yields a 20 lb or more weight-loss.

Let's move on to chapter 11, in which we discuss how to use nutritional supplements to correct lipid/lipoprotein patterns, another important component of Step 3 of your program.

Summary

- They key to exercise is to choose activities that you enjoy, or to find some means to make it enjoyable. Otherwise, you will simply find every excuse not to exercise.

- Exercise helps correct multiple lipid and lipoprotein patterns that cause coronary plaque to grow. It can also magnify the benefits you obtain through diet.

- Losing weight is most effectively accomplished through a combination of diet and exercise. *Losing* weight as opposed to *maintaining* weight requires a longer duration of exercise. Consider the use of one or more weight-loss accelerating strategies to regain control of your lipids and lipoproteins.

- Keeping count of calories you expend can be a simple though powerful method of ensuring that even ordinary activities add up to a quantity of physical effort that provides weight-control benefits.

Chapter 11

Use nutritional supplements to control plaque

Choose the right supplements to add real power to your program.

Don't underestimate the power of nutritional supplements. Just because they don't require a doctor's prescription doesn't mean they're weak or worthless.

The right supplements can pack real punch into your plaque control program. The "nutritional" tag is a misnomer that can fool you into thinking that specific therapeutic potencies are lacking. Many effective substances are classified as nutritional supplements simply because no company succeeded in obtaining patent protection as they would for pharmaceutical agents. L-arginine, DHEA, calcium pyruvate, huperzine, kava kava, and glucosamine are among agents dubbed nutritional supplements that possess specific, demonstrable therapeutic benefits. Pharmaceutical companies would have been proud to sell any of these agents if patent protection had been obtainable.

On the other hand, you could go broke buying supplements if you believed all the claims made by the supplement industry. I will tell you straight out that supplement manufacturers and distributors are guilty of making exaggerated and unsubstantiated claims over health benefits of their products. They are, after all, in the business of selling. One example of exaggerated claims made by an over-enthusiastic supplement industry is a frequent sales pitch for preg-nenolone, boasting of its purported memory enhancing effects. (Pregnenolone is a hormone that is related to testosterone, estrogen and DHEA.) This claim is based on a single study that demonstrated improved maze negotiating per-formance by—not mice, or monkeys, or humans—but *worms!* Extrapolating an observation from worms to humans is irresponsible and premature. Many clinical studies in humans are required before you begin to believe this supplement does indeed have memory enhancing effects. (By the way, there are a number of fascinating supplements that really do enhance memory, but this is a discussion for another day.) This is admittedly an exceptional example, but it illustrates just how far the industry's unrestrained enthusiasm can go.

Pick and choose the right supplements

Several supplements are broadly beneficial and nearly everyone with coronary plaque should take them. But not all supplements are for everyone. Some are helpful only to correct specific lipoprotein abnormalities. Keep in mind that supplements are just that—"supplements" to your program of nutrition principles, specific treatments and exercise, and are not meant to stand alone.

These supplements are generally safe. However, if you have a history of abnormal bleeding, a known disorder of blood clotting, stomach or duodenal ulcers, bowel dysfunction from ulcerative colitis or Crohn's disease, or a significant neurologic disorder like Parkinson's disease, you should discuss the use of any supplement with your doctor first. Always insist on an informed answer, not a flip dismissal.

If you are going to spend money on nutritional supplements, do so wisely. Spend your money on agents that provide genuine benefits. The supplements listed here are ones that I feel truly provide benefit based on both reported clinical trial data and clinical experience. No doubt, we do need more clinical data to refine our use of supplements, and to explore the effectiveness of others. Until the supplement industry matures and we gain more confidence in the health benefits of specific agents, we need to approach supplement use with a healthy dose of skepticism. That being said, I would also urge you to consider the use of the supplements listed here as powerful additions to your program that you can use with confidence.

Fish Oil (omega-3 fatty acids)

The omega-3 fatty acids (EPA and DHA) from fish oil are beneficial to anyone who has coronary plaque (calcium score >0) or has any significant lipid or lipoprotein disorder. Omega-3s reduce the release of free fatty acids from your body's fat stores. Fatty acids are the building blocks used to make triglycerides. People with high triglycerides therefore especially benefit, since omega-3s can lower triglycerides up to 50%. Omega-3s help get rid of triglyceride-rich VLDL particles. They also shift small (triglyceride-rich) LDL particles to the more favorable larger size, raise HDL modestly, and may lower Lp(a).

Just eating fish once a week may significantly lower heart attack risk, likely due to mild blood-thinning, anti-inflammatory, and inflammatory cell adhesion blocking effects. Several large studies have documented the 25–35% reduction in death from heart attack when fish is a regular part of your diet. Unfortunately, the quantity of fish you must eat to obtain *the full therapeutic benefit* in your lipoprotein patterns is unrealistic, three or four servings a day. For our purposes, a fish oil supplement is a necessity.

Of course, we want to achieve more than just lower heart attack risk. We are trying to stop the growth in plaque. For this purpose, a *minimum* of 1500 mg of the omega-3 fatty acids are required. Most fish oil capsules contain 300 mg of omega-3 fatty acids in each 1000 mg capsule. I call this a 30% preparation. (A common proportion is EPA, 180 mg, and DHA, 120 mg, for a total of 300 mg in each 1000 mg capsule, or 30%.) You can obtain a dose of 1500 mg of the omega-3 fatty acids by taking 5000 mg of fish oil, or five capsules. Some of the more concentrated (often called pharmaceutical grade) fish oils contain 50% or even up to 85% omega-3s. To determine how much fish oil to take, just add up the omega-3 component of your preparation (listed on the label) and make sure it meets or exceeds the 1500 mg per day effective doses. In general, the more concentrated, the better. Avoid cod liver oil, as it is too dilute a preparation that contains things you don't need, like saturated fats. You and your doctor may decide to use a higher dose as you assess your results. (Doses of 6000–10,000 mg/day of a 30% preparation can be safely used when triglycerides are > 400 mg/dl or VLDL is elevated.)

Fish oil is also useful to lower the blood clotting protein fibrinogen if your level is >350 mg/dl. Recall that higher levels of fibrinogen encourage blood clot formation when there is coronary plaque rupture. You and your doctor can decide if the dose of fish oil you're using is sufficient by re-checking your fibrinogen level after several weeks and increasing the dose as necessary.

Some people object to the fishy odor of fish oil capsules and the fishy belching that can follow. Refrigerating the capsules and taking them with meals can really help minimize these effects. Some preparations are worse in this regard than others and it may pay to shop around and experiment with different brands. Some manufacturers have deodorized preparations that are less fishy. Several new liquid and paste formulations are now marketed that conceal the fishy taste with fruit flavors. (See Appendix D.)

As discussed in chapter 9, the linolenic acid of flaxseed oil can also be a source of omega-3 fatty acids, but the dose required to reproduce the effects of fish oil is high and generally impractical, since the conversion of linolenic acid to EPA and DHA is inefficient. Virtually all clinical data documenting the health benefits of omega-3s has been based on fish oil sources. There is also no information examining the effectiveness of flax seed oil as a treatment for high triglycerides or VLDL. Once again, all the experience is based on fish oil. Flax seed oil is, therefore, a better adjunct to be used optionally in addition to fish oil, rather than as a replacement.

Fish oil is one of the bargains in health today. It's beneficial for a number of conditions: lipoprotein disorders, heart attack risk, cancer prevention, Alzheimer's risk, even depression, and it's inexpensive. A month's supply shouldn't cost more than $12–$15.

A very rare person will have a gastrointestinal intolerance to fish oil. Should this occur (as stomach upset, diarrhea, or excessive gas), you should discuss the continued use of fish oil with your doctor, or at the very least consider starting with a much smaller dose like 1000 mg per day and increase the dose over a several month period. People with abnormal bleeding tendencies (von Willebrand's disease, sickle cell anemia, low platelet counts, etc.) or who take the blood thinner warfarin (Coumadin) should discuss the use of fish oil with their doctor first, as fish oil does increase blood thinning modestly. Aspirin or other anti-inflammatory medicines are generally safe in combination with fish oil, but discuss this with your doctor if you have any history of bleeding or clotting disorder. In the vast majority of people, the blood thinning effect of the omega-3 fatty acids is a *benefit*, not an undesired side-effect.

l-arginine

L-arginine is an amino acid, one of the building blocks that make up proteins. L-arginine is found in many foods, particularly meats and nuts. It is truly one of the most fascinating substances available for your plaque control program.

L-arginine powerfully dilates (relaxes) the arteries of the body. In the coronaries, this discourages arterial wall injury contributing to plaque deposition and growth. Several studies document l-arginine's plaque shrinking properties. Most of these studies in humans have examined the size of plaque in carotid arteries (using ultrasound), and impressive plaque shrinkage can be achieved when l-arginine is given. In contrast, control groups not receiving l-arginine experience significant growth of carotid plaque. A similar analysis has not yet been performed in the coronary arteries. However, numerous indirect observations of l-arginine's heart effects strongly suggest that the benefits apply here, as well. People with severe coronary disease walk farther with less chest pain while taking l-arginine. Measures of artery constriction show immediate relaxation when l-arginine is administered. (Abnormal arterial constriction is very common and persistent in the presence of high blood pressure and lipid/lipoprotein abnormalities.)

One of the key ways l-arginine provides benefits is by increasing release of nitric oxide. (Not to be confused with the *nitrous* oxide, "laughing gas", given to you by your dentist for anxiety and pain relief. Despite the similar names, there is no overlap in properties.) Nitric oxide is a potent though extremely short-lived dilator of arteries, lasting only seconds after being produced in your body. The lining of artery walls is one of the major sites of nitric oxide production, where it relaxes the muscle cells that cause arteries to constrict. Because of its extremely short life, a constant supply is required to maintain relaxed arteries. Any drop in nitric oxide production (because of lack of l-arginine to fuel production, or inhibitors of the enzyme nitric oxide synthase that makes nitric oxide) and arterial tone increases and the artery constricts. The research that identified nitric oxide as an arterial dilator resulted in the Nobel Prize in 1998, awarded to Drs. Furchgott, Ignarro, and Murad.

The popular prescription medicine, Viagra, was originally intended to be a heart drug that enhanced nitric oxide production but proved more specific for the penile circulation and strengthening male erections. Nonetheless, the pharmaceutical community is very aware of the power of nitric oxide and l-arginine. Because l-arginine is a naturally occurring substance widely discussed in the scientific literature, it is not patent protectable. Products that are not patentable can therefore be sold by competitors, making development costs (hundreds of millions of dollars) difficult or impossible to recover. Pharmaceutical companies have therefore been exploring derivatives of l-arginine that are patentable. But you and I still have access to l-arginine. Once again, just because an agent does not require a doctor's prescription doesn't mean it can't be powerful and effective. Incidentally, l-arginine also has modest penile erection promoting effects, though the full benefit is rather slow to develop and may require three or so months. Future research will likely lead to pharmaceutical agents that will target nitric oxide production in specific body systems, including the coronary arteries.

Despite the abundance of data documenting l-arginine's potent effects, the dose remains somewhat uncertain. Because it is never been put through the rigors of an FDA-approval process (which requires stringent data on dosing), we need to rely on the existing data. In **Track Your Plaque,** a dose of 3000–6000 mg twice a day is recommended, best taken on an empty stomach. (The presence of other amino acids from protein foods seems to diminish the response.) For instance, if you take your l-arginine upon arising in the morning when your stomach is empty, delay breakfast for about 30 minutes. Another good time to take it is at bedtime, when your last meal was likely three hours earlier.

The dose of 6000–12,000 mg/day (3000–6000 mg twice per day) makes capsules somewhat cumbersome to use, since most capsules contain 500 mg (12–24 capsules per day!). Powdered preparations are preferable, of which several are available. You may need to shop around to find a powder you like at a reasonable price. You can generally find powdered products for around $35 for a one-pound canister. There are also some very interesting l-arginine containing products manufactured by the Cooke Pharma pharmaceutical company called Heart Bar. Though their primary product is an l-arginine containing nutritional bar, they also have a very excellent powder preparation. See Appendix D for more information on how to obtain these products.

Some people will experience loose stools when taking l-arginine, particularly at higher doses like 6000 mg per dose, occasionally even at 3000 mg. If you experience this effect, simply cut back on the dose and build up gradually over several months. This effect is generally mild (if it occurs at all) and does not lead to any long-lasting problems. If you have any active gastrointestinal diseases, particularly ones associated with diarrhea or frequent loose stools like ulcerative colitis, Crohn's disease, or malabsorption, you should discuss the use of l-arginine with your doctor before starting. L-arginine can also reactivate latent oral or genital herpes or shingles, though this is unusual. But be aware of this effect if you have a history of any of these viral eruptions, and speak with your doctor about l-arginine before starting it.

Interestingly, l-arginine is popular among anti-aging enthusiasts for its ability to provoke the pituitary gland into releasing growth hormone. Growth hormone is responsible for growth and maturation, and is believed to be responsible for the maintenance of youthful characteristics as we age. Blood levels of growth hormone drop dramatically as we age. By age 60, hardly any is produced by your pituitary. Supplemental l-arginine increases the blood levels of growth hormone, though the effect is somewhat inconsistent and variable, especially in people over age 55.

Any treatment that increases growth hormone levels can sometimes cause joint aching, and occasionally someone who is using l-arginine for purposes of inhibiting coronary plaque growth may experience some joint aching. Should this happen to you, consider stopping the l-arginine for one month, or cutting the dose in half. This effect can be from the growth hormone increasing properties of l-arginine, which can lead to a modest increase in joint fluid. Though annoying, the effect is likely harmless.

One of the difficulties in using l-arginine is that there is no quick and easy way to assess response. With niacin, for instance, we can assess your response through HDL or LDL size. With l-arginine, there are indeed ways to measure its effectiveness, but it can be painful and difficult to perform. Although l-arginine has the capacity to reduce angina (chest pain) in people with advanced coronary disease, and reduce claudication (cramping in the lower legs due to severe blockage in the leg and abdominal arteries), the great majority of participants in **Track Your Plaque** are asymptomatic. You won't, therefore, obtain relief of any abnormal heart symptom to guide you. You're left with indirect measures like blood pressure. If you start with high blood pressure, you may see a gradual drop over a period of three to six months. Some people will experience increased energy and clearer thinking. Some men will enjoy more vigorous penile erections (though not an increase in libido).

LDL lowering "adjuncts": phytosterols, oat bran, flaxseed, psyllium seed, soy protein

There are many ways to reduce LDL cholesterol and LDL particle number/apoprotein B besides prescription medicines. (In this section, for the sake of simplicity, all therapies that lower LDL can be assumed to also lower LDL particle number and apoprotein B, as well.) While these methods are not as potent as the statin drugs, they can be useful primary treatments if your starting LDL is 130 mg/dl or less. You might also consider these strategies if you are already on a medicine to reduce LDL but haven't achieved your target level. (The target LDL cholesterol for **Track Your Plaque** is 60 mg/dl.) Since these methods are commonly used along with a statin drug, I call them "adjunctive" LDL-lowering strategies. All of the adjunctive therapies listed can be used safely with any of the statin cholesterol drugs.

1) Phytosterols

Also known as stanol and sterol esters, phytosterols are derivatives of soybeans that lower LDL by binding cholesterol in the intestine, making it unavailable for reabsorption. Stanol/sterol esters are most effective when they are "esterified" and suspended in an oil base. For this reason, the phytosterols are sold as oil-based margarine or butter substitutes that taste good enough to satisfy even hard core butter lovers. The two brands presently available are Take Control Benecol, both of which you'll find in grocery stores. You can also buy non-esterified forms as powders or capsules (and therefore not suspended in an oil base), but huge quantities are required to obtain meaningful benefits, unlike the esterified form, and are therefore not recommended. Several additional esterified preparations besides butter substitutes are likely to be available in future, such as mayonnaise substitutes. The only significant downside is that, while they do indeed lower LDL cholesterol by about 10% if you use two tablespoons a day, they remain a significant calorie source. A two-tablespoon serving contains 90 calories. Otherwise, if you like to use butter or margarine, the phytosterols can be a healthy substitute. (Another choice in butter/margarine substitutes are canola-based margarines. Look for tubs rather than sticks, since the more solid stick forms have more hydrogenation. Canola margarines, of course, have the healthy monounsaturated oils and don't substantially *lower* LDL cholesterol, but instead have a neutral effect. However, the high caloric-density of these preparations is still an issue, so use these preparations sparingly.)

2) Oat Bran

Oat bran is a fabulous way to reduce LDL cholesterol. It's easy to use, is concealed easily in a variety of foods, and is effective and inexpensive. Oat bran contains abundant beta-glucan, a soluble fiber that binds intestinal cholesterol and thereby lowers blood cholesterol levels by 10–15%. Oatmeal does the same, but oat bran is more versatile and contains *twice* the amount of beta-glucan. Use two tablespoons a day in cereals, yogurt, fruit smoothies, tomato juice, etc. You can even use it heated in the microwave with water or skim milk to make a hot cereal. (Add fresh fruit, raw sunflower or pumpkin seeds, raw nuts, or dried cranberries or raisins.) A 1 lb. bag or box of oat bran often costs less than $3.00 and can be found in most grocery stores.

Oat bran is one of the few nutritional strategies that can improve the small LDL particle size abnormality. Oat bran, like raw nuts, can also serve to reduce the effective glycemic index of other foods, thereby improving your body's sugar control. This effect can cascade into improvements in HDL and triglycerides, as well as small LDL. Oat bran is so easy to use and inexpensive that it is worth including in one or more meals everyday.

3) Flaxseed

Flaxseed is among the oldest of plants cultivated by humans, with cloth woven from flax found in ancient Egyptian tombs. Flaxseed contains lignans, interesting compounds that lower LDL cholesterol and block platelet aggregation and may thereby lower heart attack risk. Several animal studies have suggested that lignans may also prevent cancer. Flaxseed is also an excellent source of linolenic acid, the omega-3 converted by the body to the omega-3 fatty acids, EPA and DHA. Two tablespoons of flaxseed contain 1.7 grams of linolenic acid.

Use flaxseed just as you would oat bran: add two tablespoons a day to yogurt, cereals, protein shakes, etc. The biggest differences are taste and price. While oat bran is nearly tasteless, flaxseed tastes nutty. It is also around two to three times greater in price. If you buy it whole and unground, grind it in your coffee grinder before use. A growing number of commercially prepared baked products with flaxseed and flaxseed oil are becoming widely available in grocery stores.

Those of you with an elevated Lp(a) might strongly consider flaxseed, as it does lower Lp(a) (though by uncertain means). Two tablespoons a day can lower Lp(a) by 7–8%. This may seem like a small benefit, but any reduction of this very stubborn abnormality is helpful.

4) Psyllium seed

Psyllium seed, better known by brand name Metamucil, is indeed helpful to promote regular bowel movements. Each individual seed is able to absorb many times its weight in water, thereby increasing stool mass. The resulting mucilaginous mass also binds intestinal cholesterol, similar to oat bran, flax seed, and phytosterols, and can lower blood cholesterol levels 10–15%.

Psyllium seed is the least versatile of our choices of adjunctive agents to lower LDL, since it can't easily be concealed in foods. Some people like the convenience, requiring little preparation beyond mixing in water or juice, and its stool bulk increasing properties. Be sure to drink extra quantities of water when you use psyllium, as it does absorb a large quantity of water in the intestine. The dose to lower LDL cholesterol is two teaspoons a day. Avoid taking vitamin supplements, especially calcium, iron, zinc, and vitamin B12, at the same time as psyllium seed, as it may bind nutrients and make them unavailable for absorption. Discuss the use of psyllium seed with your doctor before trying it if you have any history of chronic gastrointestinal disorders like ulcerative colitis, Crohn's disease, malabsorption, or have had any of your small or large bowel removed surgically.

5) Soy protein

Soy protein is among the most interesting nutritional strategies we have to lower LDL and obtain other benefits, like reduce cancer risk. Some people are wary of soy because of experiences in past with its bland taste. More recently, the current popular discussion regarding soy isoflavones, which have a phytoestrogen action, have scared men away. But, I believe that both fears are unfounded. Soy powder can now be found in many flavored varieties that conceal the bland taste, or you can easily add unflavored soy powder to other foods. The isoflavone content of soy powder is relatively small (it varies, but in the neighborhood of 100–250 mg per 25 grams). This minor quantity is commonly ingested without any evidence of adverse hormonal effects in women or men.

Soy protein is a complete protein, i.e., it has all the essential amino acids that humans require. In 1999, after an extensive scientific literature review, the FDA supported the claim that soy protein can lower cholesterol. A 25 gram serving (about three rounded tablespoons) can lower LDL cholesterol by 10% and may modestly lower triglycerides. Soy protein can be stirred into fruit smoothies and protein shakes, combined with whole grain flours to use in baking or as an egg substitute, and can be added to hot cereals. You can use other soy products like tofu (great for stir fries; tofu contains 13 grams soy protein in 4 oz), textured vegetable protein (use as a meat substitute in vegetarian chili or "meatloaf"; one burger-sized serving will provide 10 grams soy protein) and soymilk (10 grams soy protein per 8 oz glass unflavored). (See Appendix D for resources for more information on soy.) Soy powder lacks the fiber properties of flaxseed, oat bran, and psyllium seed, and so does not promote bowel health by this means. The problem with soy is acceptance. Most people just aren't too interested in trying it. But before you off-handedly dismiss the idea, soy protein is definitely worth a try. Even if you identify only one specific use that you enjoy, e.g., adding a tablespoon of soy powder to your fruit smoothie, you'll still obtain much of the benefit.

While all of the strategies in this category lower LDL, only oat bran has been shown to also increase LDL particle size, and only flaxseed and raw almonds have been shown to lower Lp(a). If you need only to lower LDL, any of these five strategies will work equally well. If you also have a small LDL particle size tendency, oat bran should be your first choice, and you can add one or two of the other adjuncts as well. If Lp(a) is among your lipoprotein abnormalities, flaxseed should be chosen first.

Not listed among the above five LDL-lowering adjunctive strategies are several other methods that also lower LDL: garlic, curcumin, green tea catechin, just to name a few. These agents tend to provide real but tiny effects that aren't very useful even as adjunctive methods to reduce LDL. They may indeed be helpful, but only to very minimal degrees. They really can't be relied on to be your primary treatment to lower LDL, nor can they be used as effective adjunctive strategies to achieve your cholesterol goal. They tend to be "fluff". Feel free to use them, but just don't expect a substantial effect. In the future, it may become possible to take specific combinations of flavonoids or to buy genetically-engineered "functional foods", such as tomatoes that are highly enriched in flavonoid content, and perhaps these may become more effective tools for us to use. But we await better information.

Raw Nuts

Raw almonds, walnuts, and pecans are packed full of healthy nutrients: monounsaturated fats, protein, fiber (insoluble), phytosterols, and even l-arginine. Walnuts, in particular, have a significant quantity of omega-3 fatty acids (as linolenic acid). Don't confuse raw nuts with salt and oil-laden nuts that are roasted in oil and canned, or dry-roasted with sugar coating ("honey-roasted") and other additives. *Raw* nuts lower LDL cholesterol, raise HDL slightly, lower Lp(a) by 8%, and blunt the blood sugar rise after meals (effectively lowering glycemic index of other foods). The benefits of raw nuts are so broad that they're recommended for virtually everyone (unless you are allergic or have a gastrointestinal intolerance). If you have high LDL cholesterol (or particle number or apoprotein B) and/or high Lp(a), raw nuts should be a part of your diet every day. Raw nuts are also strongly recommended to people with high blood sugar or borderline diabetes.

Raw nuts are especially useful to take the edge off your appetite. If you can't help overindulging at dinner, for instance, try a handful of raw nuts as a snack between lunch and dinner. Nuts are rich in fiber and healthy monounsaturated fats, and provide a sense of fullness that lasts up to eight hours. This makes you less likely to indulge in sweets and other unhealthy foods to battle hunger pangs. Calories from raw nuts can be high, however, because of the fat content. It is wise not to exceed an intake of more than ½ cup per day, or one large handful. You can usually find raw nuts at the grocery store, often in the bulk section, or you can find them in many health food stores.

Vitamin C

Vitamin C, or ascorbic acid, has been a topic of controversy for many years. There is no dispute regarding its necessity for basic health, since vitamin C deficiency causes a clear-cut and serious illness called scurvy. But the health benefits of higher doses of vitamin C have been vehemently argued for years. Conservatives argue that the replacement dose, or minimum daily requirement, of only 30 mg is required for health, with no additional benefit obtained from higher quantities. At the other end are arguments like that of Nobel laureate (for physics) Dr. Linus Pauling, who argued that mega-doses of vitamin C could cure people of atherosclerosis, based on the premise that coronary atherosclerosis represented a lesser version of scurvy. Where does the truth lie?

There's no final answer on this issue. It is worth being aware of several important observations on vitamin C. First of all, doses of vitamin C of 1000–2000 mg per day tend to modestly lower LDL cholesterol, up to 5–10 points—not a huge effect, but still a helpful addition to your program. Similar doses lower systolic blood pressure, also by a modest several points. Vitamin C has a relaxing effect on arteries, particularly if there is abnormal constriction, an effect somewhat similar to that of l-arginine (though by a different mechanism).

Does vitamin C have measurable effects on inhibiting coronary plaque growth, or reducing heart attack risk? Probably not. There have been claims made (by Drs. Linus Pauling and Mathias Rath) that mega-doses of vitamin C (up to 10 grams, or 10,000 mg) lower Lp(a) and thereby reduce plaque growth, but attempts to reproduce their efforts have been unsuccessful. Is the anti-oxidant effect of vitamin C beneficial? The answer remains unclear on this question, too. Large trials have included vitamin C as part of a mixture of anti-oxidants (often with vitamin E, selenium, and beta-carotene), and not as a single agent, and these trials have conclusively shown that combinations like this have no beneficial effects on reducing risk of heart attack. Some trials have even shown an adverse effect. The HATS trial from the University of Washington, for instance, conducted by Dr. Greg Brown, suggested that the addition of a mix of anti-oxidants obliterates the beneficial HDL-raising effects of niacin.

Some authorities have proposed that the lack of clear-cut benefit in clinical trials is due to the exclusion of other naturally occurring flavonoids that normally accompany vitamin C in whole foods. More work is needed before the answers are clear. In the meantime, the great likelihood is that vitamin C in doses of around 1000 mg per day is a good idea, with potential for modest benefits. If you have a history of kidney stones, you should not exceed a dose of 500 mg per day and should discuss this with your doctor first. Ideally, the vitamin C preparation you use should include other flavonoids, which may be listed on the label as bioflavonoid complex, hesperidin, and rutin.

Vitamin E? Tocotrienols?

Until several years ago, I advised all my patients to take at least 400 units of d-alpha tocopherol, the naturally occurring form of vitamin E. Several observational trials (i.e., studies that don't direct participants what to take) in the late 1980s and early 1990s suggested a substantial reduction in heart attack when as little as 50 units of vitamin E per day were taken. However, several subsequent well designed clinical trials ("randomized", in which participants are given vitamin or placebo without knowing which) demonstrated no cardiac benefit whatsoever from vitamin E. Many were surprised by these findings, since earlier findings suggested reduced heart attack risk with vitamin E, as well as plaque shrinkage (carotid and coronary). The message is now clear: vitamin E, even the natural d-alpha form, has no impact on reducing risk of heart attack. This does not mean, of course, that vitamin E doesn't have benefits in reducing cancer risk, Alzheimer's, or any of its other purported effects.

Interestingly, there is promising though preliminary data suggesting that the larger family of vitamin E relatives, known as tocotrienols, may significantly lower LDL cholesterol. They also provide an anti-oxidant benefit and decrease production of thromboxane, a member of the prostaglandin family of hormones that causes blood clotting. We are bound to see more data in human subjects over the next several years to help us decide whether tocotrienols are worth adding to our toolbox to control coronary plaque. But the data is too preliminary to make any decisions right now. Keep your eyes and ears open on this one.

Co-enzyme Q10

Co-enzyme Q10 (or CoQ10 for short) is another useful and fascinating substance for your **Track Your Plaque** program. It occurs naturally in the body and participates in energy generation. It is also known as ubiquinone, because of its ubiquitous presence throughout the human body. Controversies have raged over the purported anti-oxidant benefits of CoQ10, which have been observed in "test-tube" preparations but have not been fully confirmed in living humans. Claims that CoQ10 improves athletic performance have not held up well to scrutiny, as several trials have shown inconsistent effects. (Athletic performance improves in some, deteriorates slightly in others.) However, there is good evidence to suggest that CoQ10 strengthens heart muscle weakened by heart attack, viral infection, and other insults (distinct from any effect on coronary plaque growth).

For our purposes in **Track Your Plaque**, CoQ10 may help control:

Blood pressure CoQ10 has a modest blood pressure lowering effect. Doses in the range of 60–120 mg per day can lower blood pressure about 10 mm Hg, sometimes up to 20 mm Hg. Take at least twice a day (e.g., 60 mg twice a day)

Muscle aches with statin drugs The drug manufacturers of the statin drugs claim that muscle aches occur in only 2–3% of patients on any of the statin drugs to lower cholesterol (not to be confused with full-blown muscle inflammation and damage, known as rhabdomyolysis, which is rare). However, in my experience, along with many colleagues, muscle aches and mild muscular weakness occur in *30%* of people on these agents, and can develop with initiation of the drug, as well as with long-term administration. I have experienced it myself and believe it to be a real phenomenon. You find yourself less and less able to exercise and perform physically demanding activities, and begin to feel weak and drained. The statin agents deplete cellular CoQ10 and may even result in structural and biochemical changes in the mitochondria, the energy producing engines in your body's cells. Some investigators have therefore proposed CoQ10 replacement to reverse this effect. CoQ10 100 mg per day added to statin therapy frequently reduces or eliminates muscle aches and weakness within several days. This phenomenon needs to be scrutinized in a more scientific fashion, but I can strongly vouch for this effect from my own informal observations in patients and in myself. CoQ10 restores physical stamina and strength to normal within about three days. Not everyone responds, however. Three out of four people improve completely, and one out of four does not. (If you have muscle aches on your statin drug, whether or not you take CoQ10, you should still notify your physician on the small chance that actual muscle damage may be occurring, though rare.)

Lp(a) The effect is inconsistent, but CoQ10 can lower Lp(a) by up to 20% at a dose of 120 mg per day.

It is important that your CoQ10 preparation is *oil based*, i.e., CoQ10 suspended in soybean oil or other food oil, as absorption is more effective. CoQ10 is very safe and has virtually no side-effects of significance.

What supplements are *not* included

You may notice that a number of supplements that are popularly discussed in the media or supplement advertisements are not listed here: policosanol, red yeast, "no-flush" niacin, among others. However, my experience with these agents has all suggested they exert little or no effect whatsoever. I was particularly disappointed with policosanol, a sugar cane derivative that was developed and studied in Havana, Cuba. Virtually all the experimental and clinical data originates from this group of Cuban investigators, and in their reports, policosanol was tremendously effective in lowering LDL, raising HDL, lowering Lp(a), and even improving blood sugars. My experience confirmed none of these effects, at least with the preparations used.

Red yeast is a naturally occurring mixture of multiple statin agents in small quantities purported to reduce LDL cholesterol with less muscle and liver side-effects than prescribed statin drugs. Our experience with red yeast preparations, however, suggests very minimal lowering of LDL cholesterol. "No-flush niacin", or inositol hexaniacinate, is an alternative form of niacin that is supposed to avoid the warm flushing feeling that annoys some users of conventional niacin. Our experience with no-flush niacin preparations also suggest no effect whatsoever, which has been a real disappointment for the 5–10% of patients who simply are unable to achieve the dose of niacin necessary to fully correct their lipoprotein abnormalities due to this annoying effect.

Part of the problem may be that nutritional supplements are unregulated and non-standardized. It is not at all uncommon for the label to read "50 mg of—", yet have little or none of the agent at all. You could theoretically submit your supplement preparation for testing by a chemist, but this is impractical and expensive. One study of 16 brands of DHEA demonstrated that, on examination by a chemist, only *half* the bottles actually contained near the amount stated on the label. This kind of uncertainty over what you're buying will continue until either the FDA steps in to introduce formal regulation or the supplement industry itself enforces some similar oversight. However, until experience or data suggest otherwise, these preparations are not recommended.

Another group of nutritional supplements worth discussing are anti-oxidants. The list of available anti-oxidants is long. Vitamins C and E and beta-carotene (a relative of vitamin A) are anti-oxidants, as are pycnogenol, pine bark extract, grape seed extract, and lipoic acid, just to name a few. Test-tube observations have suggested that some lipoprotein particles are more susceptible to oxidation than others and can thereby be transformed into more damaging particles. Various anti-oxidant preparations do indeed, in artificial experimental settings, block damaging effects of oxidation, making LDL particles less "sticky" to the arterial wall, less likely to be ingested by inflammatory blood cells residing in the plaque, and lower abnormal arterial constriction. When scrutinized in real live humans, the benefits of anti-oxidation have not held up. Anti-oxidants can also be expensive, costing $30–60 dollars a month (each). For the time being, patience is advised until better information is available. The only exceptions are vitamin C, CoQ10, l-arginine, and flavonoids. These supplements have benefits that extend beyond the anti-oxidant question and are beneficial even though the jury is still out on their anti-oxidant effects.

If your abnormality is…then consider…

Let's summarize the possible ways to effectively use supplements according to lipoprotein abnormalities for Step 3 of your **Track Your Plaque** program. Remember, these strategies are meant to be adjunctive methods used in conjunction with diet and treatments discussed in chapter 8.

High LDL cholesterol, LDL particle number, apoprotein B—Consider oat bran, flaxseed, phytosterols (butter substitutes Take Control, Benecol), soy protein powder, raw nuts, psyllium seed (Metamucil)

Small LDL—Consider oat bran, raw almonds and walnuts; fish oil; other high-fiber sources like flaxseed, raw pumpkin and sunflower seeds.

Lp(a)—Consider flaxseed, raw almonds, CoQ10, l-carnitine, fish oil.

High triglycerides, high VLDL—Consider fish oil; raw almonds and walnuts; other high-fiber sources like flaxseed, raw pumpkin and sunflower seeds.

Low HDL—Consider oat bran, raw almonds and walnuts; fish oil.

Chapter 12

Track Your Plaque
Personal Profiles

Stories of real people in the Track Your Plaque program

Sometimes the best way to convey a message is to tell a story.

Too often, people shy away from beginning a program like this because they're afraid of what they might find, or that it might lead to frightening, risky treatments. So here are real-life profiles of several participants in **Track Your Plaque** who navigated through the process successfully. The people and stories are real but names changed to maintain privacy. Perhaps you'll see a little of yourself in these men and women.

Chris, 42 years old

Chris is a perfect example of the so-called "type A" personality: meticulous, hard-driving, always in a hurry, and a perfectionist. He started a computer consulting company while in his 30s that proved successful and sold the company several years later for a handsome profit. At this point in his life, Chris decided to find out whether the heart disease that had killed his father at age 52 was hidden inside him as well, waiting to strike. Chris was 42 years old, a husband and father of two children, eight and ten years old. He had been told repeatedly by his family physician that, given his remarkably low cholesterol values (total values of around 150–180 mg/dl; LDL cholesterol in the 70–100 mg/dl range) that he was not at risk for heart disease and that he had luckily escaped the genetics that had caused his father's heart disease.

Chris came to our center for a heart scan. His score: 104—not a disastrous score but nonetheless in the highest 10% of all men his age (90th percentile). For Chris, this was confirmation rather than revelation of something he'd suspected for several years. Chris immediately understood that he was destined to repeat his father's struggle with heart disease if he failed to take action.

The high heart scan score for age predicted a risk for heart attack of 45% over the next decade of Chris's life. He therefore sought an opinion from a cardiologist, who said, "Well, I'm not sure what that score means. In my opinion, you don't need any heart procedures, so why don't we just give you a cholesterol medicine?" The cardiologist wrote a prescription for Zocor (simvastatin, a statin cholesterol lowering drug), but Chris never filled it.

Chris was dissatisfied with this answer. He felt that it didn't make any sense to reflexively take a cholesterol lowering agent when his cholesterol was already low. He wanted to know why he had plaque in the first place. Chris heard about **Track Your Plaque** and we therefore met for consultation.

I was impressed from the start with Chris's motivation to adopt new ideas. We started with (NMR) lipoprotein assessment. As expected, his total and LDL cholesterol values were all very favorable. Here are his numbers:

Total cholesterol	152 mg/dl
LDL cholesterol	86 mg/dl
LDL particle number	1290 nm/l
HDL cholesterol	*38 mg/dl*
Triglycerides	138 mg/dl
Small LDL	*57 mg/dl*
Lipoprotein(a)	*70 mg/dl*

(The most important abnormal values are highlighted. Several other parameters not listed here were favorable, including fibrinogen and C-reactive protein.)

The cause of Chris' high score: low HDL, small LDL, and an elevated Lp(a). A cholesterol lowering statin agent may have provided some benefit, but I suggested a more specific course of therapy. Since niacin (vitamin B3) is the most potent method of both lowering Lp(a) and raising HDL, Chris was started on a prescription form of niacin (Niaspan, Kos Pharmaceuticals) that was increased over a six month period to 3000 mg per day. In addition, Chris was advised to take fish oil 4000 mg per day and l-arginine 3000 mg twice a day. Once a lover of rare steaks, Chris now followed the principles of the **Track Your Plaque** nutritional program, although he did continue to reward himself once-a-month with a filet. Chris also continued his involvement in various sports activities like basketball with friends and biking, both of which he enjoyed several times a week.

Fingerstick lipid values along the way showed a gradual increase in Chris' HDL cholesterol, suggesting that the small LDL pattern likely was responding along with it. An eventual repeat of his lipoprotein analysis six months later showed:

LDL particle number	793 nmol/l
Total cholesterol	140 mg/dl
LDL cholesterol	80 mg/dl
HDL cholesterol	60 mg/dl
Small LDL	0 mg/dl
Lipoprotein (a)	*32.4 mg/dl*

As the Lp(a) remained above our target of <30 mg/dl, testosterone cream and coenzyme Q10 was added. Chris finally achieved a Lp(a) of 24. He also added several LDL-lowering "adjuncts", including raw almonds, oat bran, and soy protein powder to lower his LDL closer to our target of 60 mg/dl.

After one year on the program, Chris's heart scan score was 121, representing a 16% increase over his prior score. Recall that, without benefit of these approaches, the average person's heart scan score increases at a rate of 30–35% per year. I explained to Chris that his 16% increase therefore represented an acceptable deceleration of his score, especially given the relatively slow-to-respond Lp(a) pattern.

Chris continued to feel well and was in the process of building another business. He stuck to his program and another year later, his heart scan score was 121, representing a 0% change from his prior score. Chris was ecstatic. With these straightforward efforts, he had managed to arrest the growth of his coronary plaque, despite having troublesome lipoprotein abnormalities. On his next scan, he was looking forward to a reduction in his score.

Track Your Plaque Suggested Lipoprotein Treatment Goals

The goals for treatment of lipoproteins can vary and are, to some degree, controversial. Nonetheless, these are the treatment goals used successfully in patients enrolled in **Track Your Plaque**. These are only *suggested* goals that may be modified to suit your particular situation, particularly the results on repeat heart scanning. This decision is best made between you and your doctor.

Parameter	Treatment Goal
LDL cholesterol	mg/dl
LDL particle number	<700 nm/l
Apoprotein B	<60 mg/dl
Small LDL	
NMR	<10 mg/dl
Electropheresis	<15% of total LDL
HDL cholesterol	>60 mg/dl
Large HDL	
NMR	>30 mg/dl
Electropheresis	>30% HDL 2b fraction
Triglycerides	<100 mg/dl
VLDL (large)	<7 mg/dl
IDL	0 mg/dl
Homocysteine	<10 mmol/l
Lipoprotein (a)	<30 mg/dl
C-reactive protein	?

(Please refer to chapter 8 for a more thorough discussion of each of the above tests.)

Deanna, 42 years old

Deanna is a 42-year-old petite, attractive mother of two, who could easily pass for someone in her mid-30s. As an exercise instructor, she is trim and muscular and accustomed to vigorous exercise, up to several hours a day.

Despite her tremendous physical conditioning, Deanna was worried that she might be destined to repeat her mom's struggle with heart disease that began with a heart attack at age 52, followed by her death at age 54. Deanna had brought this question up to her family doctor on several occasions. "You have no symptoms and your cholesterol is great. You're worrying for nothing," he'd told her. Not thoroughly convinced, Deanna underwent a heart scan to look for hidden heart disease. Her score: 275, in the highest 1% of all women her age.

Deanna came to my office, not knowing what to expect. I started by clarifying what her high score meant. First, I told her, coronary heart disease was already present and well established. Second, her heart attack risk was 4.5% per year; or 45% over 10 years—essentially a 50:50 chance by age 52. Third, if she did nothing, her score would climb 30% per year.

Deanna was stunned. Perhaps she expected me to reassure her and declare the test wrong, misleading, or silly. She broke down in tears. "I don't understand. My doctor said I wasn't even at risk for heart disease. How could this have happened? I can't possibly improve my lifestyle!"

When Deanna recomposed herself, we talked about how, in a way, this was good news. Imagine the alternatives if she'd remained unaware: suffering an unexpected heart attack in the middle of the night, being found dead by her husband or children, or developing unstable symptoms resulting in a bypass operation.

So, we discussed how this knowledge now empowered Deanna to take action. This young, apparently healthy woman had to accept that she had a dangerous level of hidden heart disease. She also would have to accommodate some changes in her life. The rewards would be substantial if we were successful: no heart attack, no bypass surgery, and no physical impairment

Deanna's lipoprotein assessment uncovered a smorgasbord of abnormalities:

LDL particle number	*1609 nm/l*
Total cholesterol	*244 mg/dl*
LDL cholesterol	*159 mg/dl*
HDL cholesterol	*46 mg/dl*
Triglycerides	112 mg/dl

(Fibrinogen, C-reactive protein, and homocysteine were favorable.)

In view of her extremely high score for a young woman, I advised Deanna to accept a vigorous course of treatment. We agreed that Deanna was to start a cholesterol medicine to lower LDL cholesterol and LDL particle number; niacin to raise HDL, correct the small LDL particle pattern, and reduce Lp(a). She added fish oil at a dose of 4000 mg per day and l-arginine, 3000 mg twice a day. She also incorporated **Track Your Plaque** nutrition principles into her diet, specifically adding raw almonds and flaxseed to lower Lp(a), as well as LDL cholesterol and particle number. Deanna adhered strictly to the program, which required several "fine-tuning" adjustments over the next several months as monitored by fingerstick lipid panels. Another full lipoprotein analysis several months later showed dramatic improvement:

LDL particle number	360 nmol/l
Total cholesterol	107 mg/dl
LDL cholesterol	37 mg/dl
HDL cholesterol	68 mg/dl
Triglycerides	37 mg/dl
Small LDL	0 mg/dl
Lipoprotein (a)	23.4 mg/dl

Deanna remained on these treatments and a repeat heart scan one year later showed an 8% increase in score, much lower than the expected 30%, representing a healthy deceleration of plaque growth. We did discuss the use of estrogen to help lower her Lp(a), but Deanna was turned-off by the potential cancer concerns and so did not include this in her program. She did agree to add l-carnitine, 1000 mg twice a day, to further lower Lp(a). After an additional year on this program, Deanna's repeat heart scan showed a score of 264, a 3% *decrease*.

Deanna has since come to terms with having heart disease. She conducts her life as usual, but has incorporated strategies to achieve control of her future health—without a surgical scar in her chest, without symptoms of heart disease, without worrying when heart attack could strike.

Esther, 67 years old

Esther is a 67-year-old grandmother of six who put a slightly different spin on **Track Your Plaque**. She differed from the usual participant in that I met her while she was experiencing anginal chest pains. Climbing stairs or walking would bring on a severe dull ache in her mid-chest. She'd recently undergone a heart catheterization performed by another cardiologist and a 90% blockage was located in the left anterior descending coronary artery, a very important artery and a very critical location. There were also several less severe plaques of 20–30% in the circumflex artery. This cardiologist advised Esther that a stent or coronary bypass operation was necessary, given the dangerous location of this blockage along with poor blood flow and chest pain symptoms. This polite, soft spoken grandmother, however, flatly refused to even consider either procedure. That's when she sought information on intensive coronary disease prevention programs.

When I first heard Esther's story, I told her that I agreed with her first cardiologist. She needed a procedure to restore flow in the artery before we could
safely proceed with any serious program of prevention. I was truly fearful for
Esther's safety. The disease in her left anterior descending coronary artery was
too far advanced and her symptoms too easily provoked for a non-procedural
approach to keep this artery from closing, which could occur abruptly at any
time. Esther's progressive symptoms suggested dangerous activity in this severe
plaque and closure could be imminent. But once again, she refused. Bad experiences of a close friend had persuaded her not to undergo any heart procedures.
I pleaded with her and even told her to get another opinion. She did, and even
this cardiologist told her that she was crazy to not have the artery fixed.

So Esther came back to my office. I reluctantly accepted that she was
absolutely and positively committed to not undergoing a procedure to fix her
blockage. We therefore began an intensive program to gain control of her
coronary disease. I asked Esther to have a heart scan. Her score:299, in the 90th
percentile for women her age (i.e., in the highest 10%). Although we already
knew she had coronary disease, the calcium score provided a starting point for
future comparison. We would try to allow as little increase in score as possible.

Lipoprotein analysis was next. Here are Esther's NMR study results:

LDL particle number	*1886 nm/l*
LDL cholesterol	*141 mg/dl*
HDL cholesterol	*40 mg/dl*
Triglycerides	97 mg/dl
Small LDL	*63 mg/dl*
Large VLDL	*82 mg/dl*
C-reactive protein	*2.2 mg/l*
Homocysteine	*23.4 mg/dl*

The causes of Esther's coronary plaque: high LDL particle number and LDL
cholesterol; low HDL; small LDL; VLDL; inflammation, as represented by an
increased C-reactive protein; and high homocysteine.

I counseled Esther on several changes in diet, particularly increasing her
intake of green vegetables and unrefined, whole foods. She loved baked foods
like cakes, pies, and cookies, which she often made for her grandchildren but
couldn't resist herself. I had to insist that she not indulge in these temptations.
I advised Esther to start a cholesterol lowering statin agent, added niacin, fish
oil 6000 mg per day, and l-arginine 6000 mg twice per day. I also asked Esther

to take folic acid 2 mg per day along with a B-complex vitamin (for vitamins B6 and B12) to lower homocysteine. She also incorporated several LDL lowering "adjunctive" supplements including oat bran, raw almonds, and ground flaxseed. Over the next several months, fingerstick lipids were used to monitor her response and niacin was increased (prescribed as long-acting Niaspan) to 2000 mg per day to increase HDL further. In the beginning, I was still very concerned about Esther's safety, so I asked that she take a platelet-inhibiting agent (Plavix) along with her aspirin to lower the likelihood of closure of the artery. We stopped this after the first six months after she'd remained without problems.

Esther's lipoprotein analysis one year later showed:

LDL particle number	877 nmol/l
Total cholesterol	151 mg/dl
LDL cholesterol	76 mg/dl
HDL cholesterol	56 mg/dl
Triglycerides	57 mg/dl
Small LDL	0 mg/dl
Large VLDL	1 mg/dl
Homocysteine	8.7 mg/dl

Contrary to my initial worries, Esther did just fine. Within two months of starting these treatments, she stopped having angina. She gradually increased her exercise and now has no angina whatsoever, even when walking her treadmill with a steep incline. A year and two months later, Esther's repeat heart scan showed an 8% increase, more than we'd like, but unquestionably better than it might have been without this approach. We then focused on ways to further increase HDL to exceed 60 mg/dl and lower LDL to our target of <60 mg/dl to achieve even better control over plaque growth.

Despite Esther's success, I would not advocate this program for people with progressive symptoms or severe blockage until they've undergone a procedure to gain stability in the arteries. (Mild blockages of less than 50% severity are indeed most likely to cause heart attack. But when a severe blockage is identified in a person with progressive or unstable symptoms, then this specific plaque may be about to close and cause heart attack. In other words, it has already ruptured.) Once you've gotten this far, as powerful as preventive therapies are, they are usually too slow to stop an artery in the process of closing. Esther, however, was an instructive exception.

Victor, 61 years old

Victor is the senior partner of the law firm he founded over 20 years ago. The firm has grown to nine partners, and Victor has borne the burden of administrative responsibilities for the group, as well as a busy personal injury law practice.

Victor's hard-working, no-nonsense approach made his law practice very successful. Despite long work hours, Victor was interested in continuing to work well beyond age 65. At 61, his wife, Liza, bought Victor a heart scan for his birthday. He balked at first, since he'd undergone stress tests every year since age 55, all normal. Victor prided himself on his good physical conditioning, maintained with a regular running program despite his long work hours.

Victor's score: 151. Not a terribly high score, but a good start to a future of heart disease, given the average rate of progression of >30% per year. I was taking care of several of Victor's wife's family members, so Liza urged Victor to come see me.

As Victor was already exercising vigorously and eating a whole food, low-fat, high-fiber diet, there was really no room to improve his excellent lifestyle. Cutting back on work stress wasn't much of an issue, since Victor enjoyed the challenges of work. We proceeded with (NMR) lipoprotein analysis. Victor's results were exceptional in that they were surprisingly bland. He had only a moderately elevated LDL cholesterol of 157 mg/dl, mildly low HDL cholesterol of 43 mg/dl, and a modest quantity of small LDL particles. I told Victor that the mild degree of his lipoprotein abnormalities was likely due to his religious adherence to an excellent lifestyle program. Had Victor not been active and been overweight instead, his score would have been far greater, or he'd have already suffered a heart attack.

I advised Victor to start a cholesterol lowering medication for his LDL, and niacin to raise HDL and extinguish the small LDL particle pattern. I asked him to add fish oil, 4000 mg per day, and l-arginine, 3000 mg twice a day. Victor proved intolerant to anything more than the starting dose of niacin (500 mg), with itching when he took more. We therefore accepted these treatments, even though his HDL increased only to 52 on the 500 mg dose.

A repeat scan one year into his program showed a heart scan score of 93—a 38% *decrease* in the first year. Victor was thrilled. Even though we had not achieved a full correction of his lipoprotein pattern, I advised him that, given the substantial drop in score, we would leave his treatments as they were and let him "coast" for the next several years while his coronary plaque regressed further.

Ed, 71 years old

Ed's story is an example of how bad a situation can get before someone recognizes that the usual answers to heart disease just don't make sense. Ed is not the typical participant in **Track Your Plaque**, since he had previously undergone bypass surgery—*four times*, in fact.

I met Ed when he was 71 years old. Ed's last bypass surgery was eight years earlier. Just in the prior year, he'd undergone four heart catheterizations with insertion of a total of seven stents into his right coronary artery and one of the bypass grafts, yet he was still having severe anginal chest pains. Minor physical efforts such as walking across a room or eating a meal provoked severe chest pain that left him exhausted for hours afterwards. He was miserable, unable to carry out even simple activities around the house. Ed was an avid golfer but was unable to play even a single hole without excruciating episodes that left him physically exhausted and emotionally demoralized.

Ed came to me for another opinion after being advised by his cardiologist that another bypass surgery was required. (By the way, I have yet to see any person survive a *fifth* bypass surgery.) Ed was understandably fed up, frustrated, and at the end of his rope. He'd heard about my program and so we sat for an hour and talked over his case. I made it clear to Ed that, at this advanced stage of his heart disease, regression of heart disease was not possible. We could at least hope for a marked slowing in the rate of his plaque growth and improvement in symptoms.

What shocked me most, however, when I reviewed Ed's prior records was that, despite two decades of conventional heart care and four bypass surgeries, he'd had his cholesterol checked only a handful of times, with the only treatment prescribed being a low dose of a cholesterol lowering drug. He'd received counseling on the usual lax diet during the cardiac rehabilitation sessions following each bypass procedure. These meager efforts constituted the full extent of the preventive strategies provided to Ed through all these crises.

Ed's case provides a good example of how it is frequently easier to get bypassed than it is to get anything more than a cursory conversation on prevention of heart disease. We started with lipoprotein testing and identified *seven* causes of heart disease that had previously gone unidentified: increased LDL particle number (despite a low LDL cholesterol), low HDL, small LDL, large VLDL, Lp(a), elevated homocysteine, and high C-reactive protein. I acquainted Ed with the **Track Your Plaque** nutrition principles, specifically concentrating on cutting back on carbohydrates because of low HDL; increased soluble fibers and other "adjunctive" strategies to decrease LDL particle number; and adding raw nuts and other monounsaturated fat sources. I also advised Ed to add niacin to lower Lp(a), raise HDL and increase LDL particle size; fish oil 3000 mg twice per day; and l-arginine 6000 mg twice a day. I also tried some unusual approaches to raise his HDL cholesterol further (he'd started with a severely low level of 24 mg/dl). Though we've managed to correct nearly all parameters to perfection, Ed still struggles to keep his HDL above 45.

(You'll recall that people with bypass grafts often cannot have a calcium score measured because of the distortions introduced by the bypass process. Scoring Ed's arteries was impossible, given his four prior bypass procedures, and a plaque score was therefore not part of Ed's program.)

Over the three years I've known Ed, he's required one procedure to stent a bypass graft. He has only occasional angina and he's now able to play a few holes of golf using a drive cart, though not a full nine holes yet. Because Ed's coronary arteries were not scorable, we really don't know how much of an effect we've had on slowing the growth of plaque. In this case, we've had to rely on a crude indicator: Ed's chest pain symptoms, which have improved dramatically.

What if we had been able to introduce these changes into Ed's life earlier, perhaps before his first bypass surgery? Of course, many of the technologies used in **Track Your Plaque** were not available 20 years ago. There are many people with Ed's future walking around now who conceivably have the power to avoid following his footsteps if the proper strategies are begun now.

Brian, 39 years old

I first spoke to Brian by phone the day after he had a heart scan at our center. I called him while on the job as the owner of a small roofing company. I don't ordinarily like to deliver upsetting news to people while they're at work, but Brian's score was alarming: 1,355—at 39 years old, this was nearly record-breaking. His score was obviously in the 99th percentile, predicting high-risk for heart attack in the next few months or years. Recall that scores of >1000 carry a *25% annual likelihood of heart attack or dying,* and risk escalates as the score climbs. This was particularly disturbing given Brian's age. He was a heart attack or bypass surgery just waiting to happen. Our initial conversation was not a pleasant one. He was caught off-guard, not expecting such a disastrous result, even though he'd seen the extensive calcium collections pointed out by the CT technologist on his scan the day before. We spoke by phone again that evening after Brian had a little while to collect his thoughts, and he then agreed to meet in consultation.

At first, I was doubtful that Brian would prove a good candidate for the program. Hard-working but also hard-living, Brian had spent his 20s and early 30s drinking and carousing, as well as working nearly 80 hours a week. His diet had been just as bad: French fries, fried chicken, bacon, fish fries, ice cream, sweets, and daily stops at fast food restaurants. In recent years, however, Brian had made efforts to lead a cleaner life for the sake of his wife and four children.

As expected, at the start of his participation, Brian's lipoproteins were awful:

LDL particle number	2386 nm/l
LDL cholesterol	167 mg/dl
HDL cholesterol	33 mg/dl
Large HDL	7 mg/dl
Triglycerides	199 mg/dl
Large VLDL	77 mg/dl
IDL	7 mg/dl
Small LDL	136 mg/dl
C-reactive protein	2.06 mg/l

What *wasn't* wrong? Based on these results, Brian was asked to follow the **Track Your Plaque** nutrition principles with a specific effort to avoid fast food. He was counseled regarding the need to avoid refined starches and replace calories with healthy oils, high-fiber foods, and lean proteins, given his low HDL cholesterol and mildly elevated triglycerides. Brian was also treated with simvastatin (Zocor), niacin (as Niaspan) 1500 mg, 4000 mg fish oil, and l-arginine 6000 mg twice a day. Correction of Brian's lipoprotein disorders to our goals required nine months, with two fingerstick lipid panels required in the interval.

To my amazement, Brian dove in to the program head-first and put forth 110% effort. He brought lunches to work rather than give in to the fast food temptation of convenience. Thankfully, Brian's wife was equally enthusiastic and changed the entire family's eating habits and food selections at home. They followed the nutrition principles and selected unprocessed, fiber-rich foods, completely eliminated fried foods and sweets, and did away with the after dinner chips and baked foods they'd indulged in every night in past. Since Brian's work was already physically demanding, he only needed to supplement his physical exertion by walking an additional 20 minutes, three times a week, and added two 15–20 minute strength-training sessions. In his first year of participation, Brian shed 24 lbs. of fat and gained 10 lbs. of muscle.

Because of his exceptionally high score, Brian also needed to have a stress test (thallium), which was normal despite the extensive plaque. Brian did require medication for blood pressure which skyrocketed when he walked a treadmill (exercise-induced hypertension), though his blood pressure has more recently improved through weight-loss efforts.

Eighteen months after our first unpleasant conversation, Brian had another heart scan. His score: 1,190—a fabulous 12% *decrease*. While his score was still high, the reduced score signified a shrinking plaque volume. With this powerful feedback, Brian is now even further energized to attain an even sharper drop on his next scan.

Several people, different stories, all successful in their own ways. I hope you see that **Track Your Plaque** is a process of self-empowerment that can give you control over plaque. It's also not that hard to follow. In the next chapter, we discuss how you can go about assembling all the pieces to put together your own **Track Your Plaque** program.

Chapter 13

Putting together your own personal Track Your Plaque program

Follow the 3 easy steps for control of your plaque

Now that it is possible to readily, easily, and inexpensively measure silent coronary plaque, there is no reason to wait for coronary disease to reach life-threatening proportions. At this point, I hope that you're eager to get underway and begin tracking *your* plaque. Where do you start? How do you assemble the pieces of the program in your city or neighborhood? In this brief chapter, we discuss the practical steps to follow to create your own personal **Track Your Plaque** program.

Putting together your own program is not tough. Taken step by step, you will likely find that one step leads logically to the next. Start with a heart scan and you will begin to understand how knowing your score crystallizes awareness of heart disease. You'll discover for yourself that just detecting plaque is not enough. It must be precisely *quantified.* The heart scan score provides an understandable, measurable, real feel for heart disease and the potential dangers ahead, far better than any other measure like cholesterol.

Once you know your score, you will want to know *why* you have plaque in the first place. That's where lipids and lipoproteins come in. Next you will want to know what to do about your plaque to keep it from growing. That is how the logical sequence of **Track Your Plaque** proceeds, as well.

Can you construct a program where you live, even if you have to travel a distance to obtain the pieces? You absolutely can. In fact, some of my patients who have participated in the program in Milwaukee have traveled from as far away as Montana, California, even New Zealand! You won't have to travel as far, since the number of scanners is booming nationwide and a scan center is bound to be within driving distance of your home. The need for a heart scan is occasional and so a scanner does not have to be in your own backyard to play a role in your program. Lipoprotein testing is getting easier and easier to obtain, as the number of physicians well-versed in this technology is rapidly growing. The lipid panels used for monitoring results along the way, and therefore required with greater frequency, can be obtained almost anywhere, even in rural areas.

Let's get started creating your own personal **Track Your Plaque**. Just follow the 3 step **Track Your Plaque** program:

Step 1—Get a coronary calcium score with a heart scan

As discussed in chapter 1, it makes no sense to pursue a program of heart disease prevention, particularly one as powerful as **Track Your Plaque,** unless you are truly at risk for heart disease in your future. You therefore need to start out by obtaining a heart scan score. Refer to Appendix B for a listing of EBT and MDCT scanners in your area. You can also find a continually updated list on the internet at www.trackyourplaque.com.

If your score is >0, coronary plaque is present and you should proceed to Step 2, lipid or lipoprotein testing, to establish the causes of your plaque. If your score is 0, meaning no detectable coronary plaque is present, no immediate action is required. Scores of 0 usually mean that your physician can address your lipids or lipoproteins just as they ordinarily would, applying standard guidelines. The intensity of therapy will likely not be as great as in **Track Your Plaque,** since your genetics and lifestyle have not succeeded in creating any measurable plaque.

Step 2—Get your lipids or lipoproteins tested

While lipid testing fails to identify the majority of people with future heart attack, it does provide a tool for treatment when plaque is established. Lipid testing is available from most physicians.

Lipoprotein testing reveals hidden causes of heart disease in 98% of people. However, despite growing popularity, lipoprotein testing has not yet been adopted by all practicing physicians. If you are interested in lipoprotein testing, start with your present doctor and ask whether he/she can provide blood drawing and interpretation services for lipoprotein analysis. If not, refer to the customer service phone numbers for the lipoprotein testing laboratories listed in Appendix C. The customer service representative for LipoScience or

Berkeley HeartLabs will be able to refer you to physicians in your area who can provide both blood drawing and interpretation of results.

If your doctor agrees to *order* the blood draw but cannot provide the service him/herself, Liposcience or Berkeley HeartLabs can direct you to designated draw sites, laboratories located nationwide that will draw your blood samples and prepare them properly. The customer service numbers listed in Appendix C can help you locate a draw site. Should you choose this route, you will still need interpretation and advice for treatment based on lipoprotein testing results. The customer service representative can help you identify a physician in your area who is familiar with the technology and may provide consultation. If you choose to use the services of a physician who is new to you, remember to first check with your insurance company to ensure that you are covered for these services ("consultation for hyperlipidemia").

Lastly, you can contact **Track Your Plaque** to provide interpretation (see Appendix C). You will still need to arrange the blood draw by one of the methods above. A detailed report will be sent to you and your doctor.

Step 3—Correct your lipid/lipoprotein abnormalities

The interpretation of your lipoprotein analysis should come with advice for treatment. Chapter 8 of **Track Your Plaque** details treatments for each specific abnormality that you and your doctor can use as a reference. Refer to chapter 9 for nutritional approaches to treat lipids and lipoproteins. Exercise tools to facilitate lipoprotein improvements are detailed in chapter 10, and nutritional supplements to help you achieve your goals are found in chapter 11.

The targets to achieve through treatment will differ when examined in light of your heart scan score. For instance, lipid results in a person with a score of 300 should be treated *differently* than another person with the same lipids but a score of zero. Suggested endpoints for therapy are discussed in chapters 8 and 13.

Those are the three simple steps of **Track Your Plaque**. Once you've successfully assembled these core pieces, you can move on to the next phase that will carry you into the future months and years.

Monitor your progress with lipids

Your physician can help decide whether your program is achieving the improvements in lipids or lipoproteins you desire. Conventional lipid analysis (total cholesterol, LDL cholesterol, HDL cholesterol, triglycerides) can be used to assess progress. When you and your physician feel that lipids have been corrected to goal, a lipoprotein analysis can be repeated to assess whether the full extent of abnormalities has been corrected. Your primary physician, the consulting physician you've chosen, or the **Track Your Plaque** consultant you use can help decide whether desired endpoints have been achieved.

Repeat your heart scan score

Consider a repeat heart scan no earlier than one year after your lipids or lipoproteins have been corrected to goal. This will usually be somewhat more than one year after your first heart scan, as lipids and lipoproteins don't get corrected immediately. It is not unusual to require several months to fully correct lipoprotein abnormalities.

If your score has not increased, congratulations! You simply need to continue your program for the next 50 years. (You will still need monitoring of lipids and liver function, when indicated, by your doctor along the way.) If there has been a large increase in score (>20%), ask your doctor to re-examine your lipid or lipoprotein analysis to identify any deficiencies in your program. The lipoprotein endpoints for treatment may need significant readjustment. If you relied only on lipids, you and your doctor should seriously consider assessing your lipoproteins, instead, to identify any hidden sources of plaque growth. You should also look objectively at lifestyle to identify any deficiencies in exercise or nutrition.

If your score increased 10–20%, you may just need to "fine-tune" your lipoprotein treatment modestly (e.g., aim for a higher HDL, lower Lp(a) further, increase fiber intake, make weight-loss a serious goal if you remain overweight, etc.) and continue for another year, at which time another heart scan score should be obtained. The process is then repeated, depending on the rate of increase of your score. Increases of <10% often decelerate further to zero-percent change or a negative change (plaque shrinkage) with time, usually another year of continuing your program "as is", or with just minor refinements.

Let's give a shove to the paradigm shift

My successful patients participating in the **Track Your Plaque** program occasionally encounter criticism from friends, family, and even physicians. Opposition to the program has included claims of not being as powerful as bypass surgery, being too slow, not scientific, too simple, or too complicated. Any new idea is likely to invite controversy, but this should spur you on to learn and understand more. I believe that much of the criticism stems from attitudes created by the huge, hungry beast that is our cardiovascular healthcare system. While the system does provide a useful service, we should try to avoid its hungry jaws with every reasonable, rational method we can get.

The tools of prevention are getting better and better. The makers of horse-drawn carriages resisted and criticized the loud, noisy, smoke-belching auto-mobile, and so will the deliverers of conventional cardiac care kick and fight to maintain their dominant role. Just as the automobile represented an inevitable evolution of technology, so too are the tools of heart disease prevention. You and I can nudge this paradigm shift by refusing to succumb to the revenue hungry jaws of the cardiovascular machine, and seize control for ourselves by applying the concepts discussed here.

Is this an end to coronary heart disease?

You have within your grasp a powerful tool that, when applied properly, has the potential to turn-off coronary plaque and drive heart attack risk down as low as possible. If everybody did this, couldn't we wipe out all coronary dis-ease? Wouldn't we be spared immense human tragedy and save huge amounts of money as a society in health care costs?

Perhaps it's too early to make such ambitious pronouncements, but I believe that the approaches discussed here do, indeed, have the potential to eradicate cardiac catastrophes for a significant segment of the population. Maybe there will come a time in the near future when the only people suffering heart attacks will be the mis-informed or non-compliant.

On the other hand, no program is foolproof and **Track Your Plaque** is no exception. Your results will depend on your dedication to nutrition, exercise, and the treatments we've discussed. Human frailty, temptation, distractions, and all the other unpredictable factors in life sometimes get in the way.

What's the most common cause for failure in our program? In my experi-ence, two areas diminish your control over plaque. One important cause is life stress, such as divorce or extreme financial struggles. No one knows why stress erodes health, but it clearly does. It elevates cancer risk, depresses immune responses, heightens inflammatory measures, as well as encourages coronary plaque growth. It also simply distracts your attention away from healthy habits. I'd love to tell you to avoid stress, but that is, of course, impossible. Stress is a part of life. If you're human, you *will* experience disappointment in your personal life and relationships, your work and career, and, unless you're among a lucky few, struggle financially from time to time. No one is spared stressful situations in life, regardless of whether you're young or old, smart or not-so-smart, thin or overweight, beautiful or not-so-beautiful, rich or poor. If stress is inevitable, the key must be in learning to deal with it. You should certainly not neglect your health program during these times, in the hopes of resuming when stress is over. Life stresses have a way of coming back. Once your recover from one stressful situation, there's often another right behind it, again threatening to erode your commitment. You've got to stick to your program, despite the distractions. It's your health and life at stake, and carrying on with your health intact and without the need for hospital catastrophe care, will, in the long run, make life more enjoyable and happier.

A second reason for failure is simply not sticking to the program. It may be insidious. You might not be fully conscious of your snacking, alcohol overuse, or neglect of physical activity. Or, you may even rationalize your way through the day, finding excuses to eat that candy bar or donut, indulge in the pizza at the dinner table, skip your walk in the neighborhood because it's cold or rainy, or you're tired. You ran out of your medicine or supplements and don't have the time to refill your supply. There's an infinite list of potential distractions that can get in our way. We all stray from perfect habits now and then; it's simply a matter of frequency and quantity. Our little indiscretions add up and the total effect can be reflected by the rate of growth of your plaque. Who knows? Maybe in 20 years there'll be some pill we can take that eliminates the need for healthy diet, exercise, supplements, etc. and you can live and eat the way you'd like. (I doubt it.) But there is certainly no such pill available now or the foreseeable future. The closer you adhere to the **Track Your Plaque** principles, the better your results will be—pure and simple.

Don't let your program end with you

Often, the best thing that comes from *your* success are the lessons you teach to your spouse, children, friends, co-workers, and others around you. They may or may not agree with the steps you take, but they will eventually recognize your success.

Some of my most gratifying patient experiences have involved identifying the silent but substantial coronary plaque in the grown children of my older patients with established heart disease. These people already know what their futures hold just by looking at their parents' lives. The **Track Your Plaque** approach crystallizes their former suspicions but provides the tools to effectively prevent following in their parents' footsteps. The 20 to 30 year advantage they have provides powerful potential to completely erase the threat of hidden heart disease.

The lessons you teach to those around you may be life-saving. Your reluctant spouse may learn how easy the program can be by watching you. He/she may still indulge in health eroding behaviors like eating badly or neglecting physical activity, but will silently observe you and realize that it's not that tough. One day, he/she may declare, "I guess I should give it a try."

Relate your experiences to others. You now know that half of all adults harbor hidden coronary plaque, and 25% of these people have extensive, potentially life-threatening plaque. Your advice is bound to hit home with at least some of the people in your sphere and perhaps trigger the proper action. If the concepts of identification and powerful prevention of heart disease disseminate widely in your family and neighborhood, maybe there'll be a day in our lifetimes when heart attack will become a rarity.

For updates, new insights, breaking research information, and practical tips on succeeding in your own personal **Track Your Plaque**, please go to our website @ www.trackyourplaque.com. We also want to hear your story. Please e-mail us at the above website. Good Luck!

Appendix A
A Review of the Scientific Evidence

The Use of Calcium "Scoring" as a Surrogate Marker
for Coronary Artery Disease

Here we review the background scientific evidence that supports the concept of coronary calcification "scoring" as a means to measure coronary plaque. This discussion is meant for both the professional as well as the interested non-professional reader to gain a better understanding of the substantial evidence documenting this approach. We will discuss how coronary calcium predicts future coronary events and how score reduction suggests a markedly reduced risk. Because of the volume of data that has been generated on this technology and its applications, our discussion will be confined to those issues relevant to the calcium score as a surrogate measure of coronary disease in *asymptomatic* persons.

Severity of stenosis is a poor predictor of future myocardial infarction

Conventional diagnostic testing for coronary disease is intended to identify atherosclerotic stenoses sufficient to reduce coronary blood flow and generate myocardial ischemia. Thus, stress testing in its various forms are simply provocative maneuvers that induce ischemia during periods of increased myocardial energy demands. The identification of myocardial ischemia is, therefore, often equated in clinical practice with the presence of coronary disease.

However, the premise that coronary events are predicted by only severe (>50% diameter reduction) stenoses has been challenged by several angiographic studies that demonstrate that as many as 70% of all acute coronary events develop from "mild" (<50% diameter reduction) coronary stenoses.[1-3] Yet mild stenoses are not generally detectable by stress testing, nor do they provoke cardiac symptoms.

Other lines of evidence have suggested that the most powerful predictor of future coronary events is the presence of atheromatous plaque[4], or coronary "plaque burden"[41], irregardless of severity of stenoses. The more extensive the plaque, the greater the future risk of infarction and death.

A method to quantify atherosclerotic coronary plaque would conceivably provide a superior measure of future coronary events. The greater the quantity of plaque, the higher the coronary event risk, even without ischemia and in the absence of symptoms. Ideally, this method should be accurate, reproducible, safe, and inexpensive. It would also be quantitative, potentially allowing tracking over time to establish progression and heightened event-risk, or regression with a reduction in event-risk.

Calcium accompanies atherosclerotic plaque

The development of atherosclerotic plaque in the coronary arteries proceeds through a series of predictable stages from adolescence to adulthood. For many years, it has been recognized that calcium can occur as part of the atherosclerotic process, though it was initially felt to accompany only more advanced phases of the disease.[5] However, more recent observations have identified calcium at a relatively early point in the growth of atherosclerotic plaque. Similar to the calcium found in bone, calcium in coronary plaque occurs as hydroxyapatite.[6] Rumberger et al[7] clarified the quantitative relationship of calcium and coronary plaque by demonstrating that calcium follows a consistent, linear relationship with the cross-sectional area of atherosclerotic plaque. In this histopathologic study, calcific components constituted approximately 20% of plaque area, and this proportion held consistent in all three coronary arteries with examination of males and females, younger and older, and in persons with and without manifest clinical evidence of coronary disease.

Because of the consistent proportion of calcium to plaque, Rumberger et al proposed that calcium be used as a "surrogate" measure of coronary plaque burden.

Calcium is accurately measured using electron-beam tomography (EBT)

The "ultra-fast" CT scanner, or EBT, permits precise quantification of coronary calcium. Calcium is radiographically-dense and can be readily visualized in the axial sections generated by EBT or CT scanners. However, the slow speed of image acquisition by earlier generations of CT scanners (around 1000 msec per image) does not permit clear visualization of calcium in coronary plaque due to coronary motion. The EBT device obtains images in 100 msec. or less with sufficient temporal and spatial resolution to reliably visualize moving coronary arteries. With this imaging technology, visualization of calcium in young people with only small quantities of calcium, even in the absence of angiographic stenosis, is possible.

The fastest of the new "multi-detector" helical and spiral scanners, which use multiple detecting rings to partially circumvent the need to rotate a full 360-degrees around the patient, may achieve scan times of 250–300 msec., approaching the 100 msec scan speed of the EBT device (discussed further below).

Janowitz et al[8], Simons et al[9], and Detrano et al[10] have confirmed that coronary calcium as measured by EBT correlates well with the amount of calcium found on histopathologic analysis (r = 0.95–0.97). These and other investigators have concluded that EBT coronary calcium measurement is therefore a reliable measure of plaque burden. These same studies, however, did also point out that calcium measurement by EBT or by direct pathologic examination, correlated only moderately with stenosis severity.

Coronary calcification—Scoring methods

The most widely used method to quantify coronary calcium by EBT is the approach introduced by Agatston.[14] The area of calcified plaque (in mm^2) on the axial CT image is multiplied by a coefficient based on radiographic density as expressed in Hounsfield units. The greater the radiographic density of the calcified plaque, the greater the coefficient. For a density of 0–130 the coefficient is 0; for 130–200, the coefficient is 1; for 201–300 the coefficient is 2; for 301–400 the coefficient is 3, and for >400 the coefficient is 4. Several investigators have reported large series of patients undergoing EBT[15–17] that have consistently shown the correlation of a graded pattern of increasing scores in men and women with advancing age. Calcified plaque generally begins to be detectable in men beyond age 35 years, with a rapid increase in prevalence over age 40. In women, scores >0 generally appear beyond age 45 with the same rapid increase in prevalence at age 55. Score distribution can be stratified by age and expressed as quartiles of score, or "percentile rank". The prevalence of calcium by EBT increases with age such that, at age 65, for instance, the score representing the 50th percentile in men is 201.

The reproducibility of calcium by EBT has been questioned in past due to several reports of variation in scoring as high as 40–50%. However, with more recent scanners and improved scanning algorithms, reproducibility has been improved.[18] Studies examining the timing of slice acquisition with regards to the electrocardiographic QRS-complex have especially reduced variation in scoring due to cardiac motion. Earlier studies used a QRS-complex triggering time of 80% of the R-to-R interval. More recent studies have demonstrated that slice acquisition at 30–50% of the R-to-R interval (during isovolumic relaxation of the ventricles) has minimized cardiac motion, reducing variability in scoring.[19] One quirk in the arithmetic of examining scan reproducibility is that at lower scores, a small absolute difference could represent a large percentage change. For example, a score of 4 that, when repeated, is re-scored as 6, represents a 50% difference, though the absolute difference is a relatively small 2. On the other hand, a score of 1004 followed by a repeat score of 1006, despite having the same absolute difference, will show a minor (<1%) variability by percentage. The mathematical distorting effect that depends on the magnitude of the initial score needs to be taken into consideration when examining questions of reproducibility. This effect was well demonstrated by the analysis of Achenbach et al[18]. Using an Imatron C–150 scanner with half the patients scanned at 40% of the R-to-R interval, variability of scores below 100 was 42%, while variability of scores >100 was 10.5%.

Callister et al[20] developed a modified scoring process that uses a plaque volume-measuring (volumetric) approach, rather than the area and density-coefficient method of Agatston. This approach incorporates a slice-to-slice mathematical smoothing algorithm using isotropic interpolation that is less affected by partial volume averaging effects and has reduced variability to 7.8%. Callister et al have also proposed that volumetric measures of plaque may prove more useful when trying to achieve regression of plaque, since regression results in a shrinking plaque volume and area but a potential increase in calcium density. Use of the Agatston score, representing a combination of area and density, would therefore be distorted by a decrease in one parameter and increase in the other. A volumetric measure, on the other hand, might more accurately reflect the plaque-shrinking effect of therapy. Comparisons of the volumetric vs. the Agatston methods for this purpose need to be further examined.

Correlation of coronary calcium score, stenosis severity, and myocardial ischemia

Many earlier investigations of calcium scoring focused on how well calcium scores correlated with angiographic measures of stenosis severity. The data were consistent in suggesting that the greater the calcium score, the more likely that significant stenoses (usually defined as greater than 50% diameter reduction by angiography) would be present. However, the relationship of calcium score with stenosis severity is weaker than its relationship with atherosclerotic plaque area. In general, EBT calcium scoring is highly sensitive for detecting angiographic stenoses >50%, but lacks specificity. In Haberl et al's[17] comparison of coronary angiography and EBT calcium scoring in 1,764 patients (1,225 men, 539 women), a calcium score of 0 was associated with an extremely low likelihood of stenosis (<1%). In men, calcium scores at the >20th, >50th, or >75th percentile yielded sensitivities to detect angiographic stenoses of 97%, 93%, and 81%, respectively. In women, sensitivities were 98%, 82%, and 76%, respectively. Specificity was 77% in both men and women. In other words, the presence of any calcium represented by a score >0 was very sensitive for the presence of any angiographic stenosis, but only moderate specificity. Overall, a calcium score in the 75th percentile carried a 77% likelihood of a stenosis >50%.

Budoff et al[21] similarly reported on a multi-center trial involving 710 patients. Calcium scoring yielded a sensitivity of 95% for detecting angiographic stenoses (>50%) with a specificity of 44%. A meta-analysis of nine studies involving 1,662 patients reported similar findings, with a sensitivity of 92.3%, specificity of 51.2%.[22]

Rumberger's[7] histopathologic analysis of coronary arteries suggest an explanation for the discrepancy between this measure of plaque burden and stenosis severity. This analysis demonstrated that, while calcium area correlated very well with plaque area, plaque was often accompanied by enlargement of the artery diameter, thus preserving the internal diameter of the vessel. This appeared to be consequent to "adaptive remodeling", i.e, compensatory enlargement of the arterial diameter in segments of the artery wherein plaque accumulates, consistent with the principle first proposed by Glagov[40] based on pathologic examination of coronary arteries. In other words, the presence of calcium was a reliable measure of plaque but, because of compensatory artery enlargement, or remodeling, it correlates less well with stenosis severity. For these reasons, calcium scoring can be regarded as an excellent indicator of plaque burden, but only a moderately reliable indicator of angiographic stenosis severity.

Accordingly, we should not expect stress testing to correlate perfectly with coronary calcium, either, since the various stress test modalities are designed to identify ischemia, not plaque. He et al[23] provided the clearest experience on this question. They studied 411 asymptomatic subjects (79% male) with both EBT calcium scoring and stress thallium. Higher calcium scores were increasingly likely to be associated with stress perfusion abnormalities. No subject with a score of 0–10 had a perfusion abnormality; calcium scores 11–100 yielded a 2.6% likelihood of a perfusion abnormality; calcium scores of 101–399 had an 11.3% likelihood of a perfusion abnormality; and calcium scores of 400 or greater yielded 46% with a perfusion abnormality. These findings suggest that as EBT calcium score increases, the probability of ischemia also increases. The majority of people with a calcium score >0 will therefore have a negative stress test, i.e., the presence of plaque is not associated with ischemia. Note that the likelihood of an abnormal stress thallium at a score of 400 is only 46%, yet extensive plaque is present, consistent with the known low sensitivity of stress testing for coronary plaque.

How good a predictor of coronary events is coronary calcium in the *absence* of myocardial ischemia? We next discuss the value of coronary calcium scoring as a predictor of events in asymptomatic persons.

Coronary calcium predicts coronary events

If coronary calcium correlates with the extent of plaque, then the calcium score should be predictive of coronary events. This issue has been examined in several trials and, in fact, calcium scoring has proven to be a very powerful predictor of future coronary events. This holds true even in the absence of symptoms.

Arad et al[24] followed 1,173 asymptomatic patients for a mean period of 3.6 years and in whom no therapeutic interventions were made after an EBT scan. 39 coronary events (death, myocardial infarction, and coronary revascularizations) were observed over the follow-up period. The odds ratio for a calcium score >160 was 15.8 for any coronary event (including revascularization), 22.2 for a "hard" coronary event (non-fatal myocardial infarction or death). (The authors state that the study was designed such that the calcium score did not enter into clinical decision making.)

Raggi et al[15] prospectively followed 632 asymptomatic patients (50% men) referred for EBT scanning because of the presence of coronary risk factors. Over the average period of follow-up of 32 months, the number of "hard" events (death and non-fatal myocardial infarction) in the highest quartile of calcium score was 20 times higher than that of the lowest quartile. In comparison, risk factors (considered alone, without calcium score) in the upper quartile had six times greater events than the lowest quartile. The annualized event rate and odds ratios for each of the four quartiles of calcium score are shown in the table below:

Quartile	Annualized Event Rate		Odds Ratio	
	Calcium Score	Risk Factors	Calcium Score	Risk Factors
1st	0.2%	0.5%	1.0	1.0
2nd	0.2%	1.4%	1.0	3.1
3rd	1.4%	1.4%	6.2	3.1
4th	4.5%	3.1%	21.5	7.0

Adapted and modified from Raggi et al[15]

These data suggest that calcium scores are a powerful predictor of coronary events, with greater ability to predict events than conventional risk factors. Note that calcium score in this analysis also more effectively distinguished low-risk (1st quartile) from high-risk (4th quartile). A similar distinction was made by risk factors, but not as dramatically. The odds ratio of 21.5 in the highest quartile of calcium score compared with the odds ratio of 7 for risk factors suggests that a high calcium score carries great discriminatory value in identifying patients likely to suffer a future coronary event. Raggi et al point out that, in this study, 70% of all patients with cardiac events were in the 4th quartile of calcium score (75th percentile); 85% of all events were in the 3rd and 4th quartile (50% percentile and greater). In other words, the 3rd and 4th quartile of scores (equal to or greater than the 50th percentile) identified 85% of people destined to suffer a future major cardiac event.

Wong et al[25] reported similar findings in a cohort of 926 asymptomatic subjects (735 men, 191 women). At baseline, 60% of men and 40% of women had a calcium score >0. Over a mean follow-up period of 3.3 years, the relative risk of cardiovascular events (myocardial infarction, death, revascularization) for scores of 81–270 was 4.5; relative risk for scores >271 was 8.8. There were no events in persons with scores of 0.

A larger study by Kondos et al[43] followed 5635 subjects with ages ranging from 30 to 76 years after EBT scan for three years. Calcium score and percentile rank proved superior predictors of cardiac events compared to conventional risk factors, with relative risk of 10.5 in males, 2.6 in females. Greenland[44] et al demonstrated that calcium scores add important prognosticating information to the calculated Framingham risk calculation, particularly those in the intermediate risk category (calculated coronary event risk 10–20% over 10 years). For instance, for persons designated as intermediate risk by Framingham, a calcium score of 80 or greater predicts that the risk is actually three-fold higher than predicted by risk factors alone.

The predictive power of calcium scores was very dramatically illustrated by the report of Wayhs et al[26]. Ninety-eight asymptomatic persons (average age of

62 years) with high calcium scores of >1000 were identified who did not immediately undergo any cardiac testing or intervention, including stress testing. Subjects were followed for an average of 17 months after their scan. Over this relatively brief period of time, 35 subjects (36%) died or suffered a myocardial infarction. The annualized event rate for subjects with scores >1000 was an extraordinary 25%.

Direct comparisons of stress testing and calcium scoring for prediction of cardiac events in *asymptomatic* persons are not presently available. However, several studies have demonstrated that stress testing in asymptomatic populations is plagued by a high false-positive rate for predicting hard coronary events (death, myocardial infarction), with positive predictive values of <10%.[49, 50] A follow-up study of the Lipid Research Clinics cohort of 2,994 asymptomatic females showed that ST-segment changes (as much as 2 mm ST-segment depression) were *not* predictive for cardiac events over the 20 years of the study.[51] The usefulness of coronary calcium scoring to predict events in asymptomatic populations may prove a very useful application, given the pitfalls of stress testing.

Despite the present lack of comparative data, it is quite clear that calcium scoring identifies coronary plaque and provides graded prediction of risk, even in asymptomatic populations. One of calcium scoring's most attractive features is its *quantitative* nature: low scores predict lower risk, intermediate scores predict intermediate risk, and high scores predict higher risk. Data such as that reported by Arad et al[24] and Wayhs et al[26] suggest that the calcium score has potential to accurately identify the especially high-risk *asymptomatic* patient with far greater reliability than stress testing.

Who should be scanned?

Though this appears at first to be a simple question, it is probably among the most difficult of issues surrounding sub-clinical plaque detection, and carries the greatest potential financial impact. If cost were not an issue, then widespread screening could be more readily advocated. Broad, unselected screening of asymptomatic people carries the greatest chance of identifying those at risk of future coronary events, but introduces higher costs and some exposure to radiation. On the other hand, an excessively restrictive selection process would miss many potential people at risk. Some have advocated using conventional coronary risk factors (lipid parameters, hypertension, diabetes, family history) to determine who may be appropriate for coronary calcium scanning. But it is quite clear that risk factors fail to predict approximately half of all future cardiovascular events[29], and would therefore be overly restrictive.

Hecht et al[30] has argued persuasively on the pitfalls of using lipid parameters to select persons appropriate for heart scans. 931 consecutive asymptomatic, self-referred persons presenting for EBT heart scans underwent simultaneous fasting lipid examination. People being treated for any hyperlipidemia were excluded, as were those with a history of clinical coronary disease. Hecht et al found that total cholesterol, LDL cholesterol, HDL cholesterol, the total cholesterol to HDL ratio, and triglycerides did not reliably predict the presence or absence of plaque as judged by calcium score. For instance, at a level of LDL >130 mg/dl, 53% of participants had an abnormal calcium score (>0), 47.0% had a negative score. The lack of correlation was found when using calcium score percentile rank, as well. The combination of LDL<130 mg/dl and HDL >35 mg/dl, generally regarded as a low risk group, was associated with a 50% incidence of coronary calcium. Conversely, 32.6% of subjects with a "high-risk" LDL of >160 mg/dl had calcium scores of zero. It was therefore concluded that lipid parameters could not be used to reliably identify who was likely to have or not have coronary plaque as measured by EBT.

The analysis of Hoff et al[16] described the distribution of EBT calcium scores in over 35,000 subjects ranging in age from 30 to 76 years old. This population was self-selected, primarily white, and 74% men; all scanning was performed at the University of Illinois-Chicago. Distribution of scores by age show that significant numbers of subjects in the 75th percentile or greater for calcium scores (a higher risk sub-group) begin to appear in substantial numbers over age 40 in men, over age 50 in women. These observations have provided the basis for many scanning centers recommending calcium screening for men over 40, women over 50. How these age-dependent cut-offs should be combined with risk factors still remains unsettled.

While more investigation is required, a growing practice in many centers is to screen people by age only, without consideration of risk factors, given the deficiencies of risk factors in selecting those truly at risk for a coronary event. Grundy[31] has argued that calcium score be used to replace age as one of the risks for coronary events.

MDCT: an emerging technology

Coronary calcium scoring has traditionally been performed on EBT devices because of the speed of image acquisition. Coronary motion during the cardiac cycle tends to blur images if acquisition extends into ventricular systolic contraction or relaxation or atrial contraction. The time window of opportunity is therefore somewhat narrow. The original axial CT scanners acquired images in approximately 1000 msec (the duration of a full cardiac cycle at a heart rate of 60 bpm), making coronary calcium visualization virtually impossible. The advent of "spiral" and "helical" technologies, in which the x-ray gantry rotates around the patient, has shortened the time required. However, the development of multiple detector rings, such that several simultaneous images can be obtained in a single gantry rotation, has considerably improved temporal resolution. In a 16-slice multi-detector CT (MDCT) device, effective scan time is around 250 msec. Data suggest that MDCT scanning at this speed provides scoring data similar to that of EBT.[45] The radiation dose with a 4-slice or greater MDCT scanner is equivalent to that during EBT, provided the cardiac cycle is prospectively gated.[46]

Coronary calcium increases

If calcium scoring is indeed a surrogate measure of plaque volume, we should expect that it increases in predictable fashion as disease progresses, and indeed it does. However, the magnitude of increase surprised most observers when first reported by Janowitz et al.[32] In this early report, 25 subjects underwent serial EBT scans 13 months apart. Ten of the subjects had also undergone coronary angiography for symptoms of heart disease. The symptomatic subjects experienced a calcium score increase of 48% over the 13 months. The remaining asymptomatic subjects showed a 22% increase. While the distinction of symptomatic vs. asymptomatic may be somewhat arbitrary, the rapidity of increase even in the asymptomatic group was substantial.

Maher et al[33] described a series of 81 patients (45 men, 36 women) who underwent serial EBT scans over a mean interval of 3.5 years. Participants were selected without knowledge of risk factors or coronary disease status. The annual rate of increase in calcium score was 24%. In a similar experience with 299 subjects, Budoff et al[34] observed a 33% annual rate of increase in calcium score.

Previous angiographic studies have demonstrated increasing risk for major cardiac events with progressive angiographic severity of coronary disease.[47, 48] Evidence is also accumulating that suggests that an increase in calcium score predicts a much heightened risk for coronary events. Conversely, stable or decreasing scores (on statin therapy) appear to carry a sharply reduced risk of events. Raggi et al[35] reported an experience with 269 asymptomatic patients who underwent sequential EBT scanning. Over a 2.5-year follow-up period, 25 cardiac events occurred (16 revascularizations and 9 deaths and non-fatal myocardial infarctions). Of these 25 events, 23 (92%) occurred in the individuals who showed progression of coronary calcification; only 2 of the events occurred amongst patients with stable or reduced scores. The average rate of progression in patients with events was 40%, compared to 22% in those without events.

Shah et al[36] reported a similar experience in 225 patients with serial EBT scans over a three-year average period of follow-up. Eight myocardial infarctions and 18 coronary revascularizations occurred. Patients having events had an average score increase of 78% over the period of follow-up, compared to 37% in those without events. Most notably, *no events occurred in patients with stable or reduced scores*. The odds ratio for an event with calcium score increase >20% per year was 14.6.

Coronary calcium can be reduced

If the coronary calcium score can be used quantitatively to identify the presence of coronary plaque and tracked to measure progression, then it would be only reasonable to suspect that the same measure might be used as a method to track regression, i.e., calcium score reduction.

The first report of such an application of calcium scoring was by Callister et al[37], in which 149 patients referred for EBT scoring by their primary care physicians were followed for one year. No specific therapy was instituted, but was left to the discretion of the referring primary care physician. After one year, an EBT scan was repeated. Patients who received treatment with a statin agent had an average increase in score of 5%. In contrast, patients who received no statin therapy had an average rate of increase of 52%. Interestingly, the majority of patients who had LDL cholesterols lowered to <120 mg/dl had an average *reduction* of 7% in score, i.e., presumed regression of coronary plaque.

Budoff et al[34] observed a similar pattern in 299 asymptomatic patients followed for up to 6.5 years. While the group as a whole experienced a 33.2% annual rate of increase in calcium score, persons treated with a statin agent demonstrated an average annual rate of increase in calcium score of 15%, while untreated patients had a 39% rate of annual increase. Treatment was not prospectively controlled and therefore not conducted to achieve specific therapeutic end-points.

Achenbach et al[38] reported results of a prospective trial of treatment with cerivastatin (0.3 mg/day) in 66 patients who had an initial baseline EBT calcium score >20 and an LDL cholesterol >130. The baseline scan was followed by one year of no therapy and then a repeat scan. Treatment with cerivastatin was then initiated and a third scan was obtained at the end of another year. Cerivastatin lowered mean LDL from 164 mg/dl to 107 mg/dl. During the first year without treatment, the median annual increase in calcium scores was 25%. During the subsequent treatment period, the median rate of increase was 8.8%. In a subset of patients who achieved LDL cholesterols of <100 mg/dl during treatment, the median relative change was 27% during the initial untreated period,–3.4% during treatment, i.e., presumed regression was achieved when LDL was treated to <100 mg/dl. Unfortunately, the trial size was limited by the recall of cerivastatin by its manufacturer.

One unexplored area is the effect of combination therapy on coronary calcium score. The HATS trial[39] demonstrated a reduction in relative risk of events of 90% on combination therapy (niacin + simvastatin) compared to placebo. Angiographic regression of disease was also seen on combined therapy. Though this was an angiographic trial, we might reasonably extrapolate this important experience to calcium scoring and expect that reductions in score on combination therapy will likely exceed that seen with statin therapy alone.

Conclusion

Coronary calcium scoring provides a safe, reliable, and inexpensive method to identify coronary plaque. The calcium score quantifies coronary plaque burden and correlates well (especially as percentile rank) with risk of future coronary events, even in the absence of symptoms. Because the calcium score is a quantitative measure of plaque, it is also a promising tool to assess disease progression, stabilization, or regression. It is in this area that the most exciting applications of calcium scoring have yet to be realized. Further study is needed to explore how calcium score might be used as an endpoint of therapy, as a measure not only of plaque volume but also a surrogate measure of plaque "inactivation", i.e., regression of internal plaque activities (e.g., inflammation, metalloproteinase activity) that lead to acute coronary events. Existing data suggest that stabilization of calcium score or score reduction is associated with a dramatic decrease in risk of coronary events. To date, the clinical evidence strongly points toward LDL cholesterol lowering via statin therapy as a means to achieve coronary calcium score reduction. Future clinical trials will need to examine how combination therapies (e.g., statin + niacin) will impact on calcium score and event risk.

References:

1 Ambrose JA, Tannenbaum MA, Alexopoulos D, Hjemdahl-Monsen CE, Leavy J, Weiss M, et al. Angiographic progression of coronary artery disease and the development of myocardial infarction. J Am Coll Cardiol 1988;12:56-62.

2 Little WC, Constantinescu M, Applegate RJ, Kutcher MA, Burrows MT, Kahl FR, et al. Can coronary angiography predict the site of a subsequent myocardial infarction in patients with mild-to-moderate coronary artery disease? Circulation 1988;78:1157-1166.

3 Giroud D, Li JM, Urban P, Meier B, Rutishauer W. Relation of the site of acute myocardial infarction to the most severe coronary arterial stenosis at prior angiography. Am J Cardiol 1992;69:729-732.

4 Kuller LH, Shemanski L, Psaty BM, Borhani NO, Gardin J, Haan, MN, O'Leary DH, et al. Subclinical disease as an independent risk factor for cardiovascular disease. Circulation 1995;92:720-726.

5 Blankenhorn DH, Stern D. Calcification of the coronary arteries. Am J Roentgen 1959;81:772-7.

6 Fitzpatrick LA, Severson A, Edwards WD, Ingram RT. Diffuse calcification in human coronary arteries: association of osteopontin with atherosclerosis. J Clin Invest 1994;94:1597-1604.

7 Rumberger JA, Simons DB, Fitzpatrick LA, Sheedy PF, Schwartz RS. Coronary artery calcium areas by electron beam computed tomography and coronary atherosclerotic plaque area: a histopathologic correlative study. Circulation 1995;92:2157-2162.

8 Janowitz WR, Agatston AS, Kaplan G, Viamonte J Jr. Differences in prevalence and extent of coronary artery calcium detected by ultrafast computed tomography in asymptomatic men and women. Am J Cardiol 1993; 72:247-254.

9 Simons DB, Schwartz RS, Edwards WD, Sheedy PF, Breen JF. Noninvasive definition of anatomic coronary artery disease by ultrafast computed tomographic scanning: a quantitative pathologic comparison study. J Am Coll Cardiol 1992;20:1118-1126.

10 Detrano R, Tang W, Kang X, Mahaisavariya P, McCrae M, Garner D, et al. Accurate coronary calcium phosphate mass measurements from electron beam computed tomograms. Am J Cardiac Imag 1995; 9:167-173.

11 Budoff MJ, Mao S, Zalace CP, Bakhsheshi H, Oudiz RJ. Comparison of spiral and electron beam tomography in the evaluation of coronary calcification in asymptomatic persons. Int J Cardiol 2001;77:181-188.

12 Carr JJ. Coronary calcium: The case for helical computed tomography. J Thoracic Imaging. 2001;16:16-24.

13 Rumberger JA. Noninvasive coronary angiography using computed tomography. Ready to kick it up another notch? Circulation 2002;106:2036-2038.

14 Agatston AS, Janowitz WR, Hildner FJ, Zusmer NR, Viamonte M Jr, Detrano R. Quantifiction of coronary artery calcium using ultrafast computed tomography. J Am Coll Cardiol 1990;15:827-832.

15 Raggi P, CallisterTQ, Cooil B, Zuo-Xiang H, Lippolis NJ, Russo DJ, Zelinger A, Mahmarian JJ. Identification of patients at increased risk of first unheralded acute myocardial infarction by electron-beam computed tomography. Circulation 2000;101:850-855.

16 Hoff JA, Chomka EV, Krainik AJ, Daviglus M, Rich S, Kondos GT. Age and gender distributions of coronary artery calcium detected by electron beam tomography in 35,246 adults. Am J Cardiol 2001;87:1335-1339.

17 Haberl R, Becker A, Leber A et al. Correlation of coronary calcification and angiographically documented stenoses in patients with suspected coronary artery disease: results of 1,764 patients. J Am Coll Cardiol 2001;37:451-457.

18 Achenbach S, Ropers D, Mohlenkamp S, Schmermund A, et al. Variability of repeated coronary artery calcium measurements by electron beam tomography. Am J Cardiol 2001;87:211-213.

19 Lu B, Mao SS, Zhuang N, et al. Coronary artery motion during the cardiac cycle and optimal ECG triggering for coronary artery imaging. Invest Radiol 2001;36:250-256.

20 Callister TQ, Cooil B, Raya SP, Lippolis NJ, Russo DJ, Raggi P. Coronary artery disease: improved reproducibility of calcium scoring with an electron-beam CT volumetric method. Radiology 1998; 208:807-814.

21 Budoff MJ, Georgiou D, Brody A, Agatston AS, Kennedy J, et al. Ultrafast computed tomography as a diagnostic modality in the detection of coronary artery disease: a multicenter study. Circulation;1996;93:898-904.

22 Nallamothu BK, Saint S, Bielak LF, et al. Electron-beam computed tomography in the diagnosis of coronary artery disease: a meta-analysis. Arch Intern Med 2001;161:833-838.

23 He Z, Hedrick TD, Pratt CM, Verani MDS, Aquino V, Robert R, Mahmarian JJ. Severity of coronary artery calcification by electron beam computed tomography predicts silent myocardial ischemia. Circulation 2000;101:244-251.

24 Arad y, Spadaro LA, Goodman K, Newstein D, Guerci AD. Prediction of coronary events with electron beam computed tomography. J Am Coll Cardiol 2000; 36:1253-1260.

25 Wong ND, HSU JC, Detrano RC, Diamond G, Eisenberg H, Gardin JM. Coronary artery calcium evaluation by electron beam computed tomography and its relation to new cardiovascular events. Am J Cardiol 2000;86:495-498.

26 Wayhs R, Zelinger A, Raggi P. High coronary artery calcium scores pose an extremely elevated risk for hard events. J Am Coll Cardiol 2002;39:225-230.

27 Hachamovitch R, Berman DS, Kiat H, et al. Exercise myocardial perfusion SPECT in patients without known coronary artery disease: incremental prognostic value and use in risk stratification. Circulation 21996;93:905-914.

28 Iskander S, Iskandrian AE. Risk assessment using single-photon emission computed tomographic technetium-99m sestamibi imaging. J Am Coll Cardiol 1998;32:57-62.

29 Wald NJ, Law M, Watt HC, Wu T, Bailey A, Johnson AM, Craig WY, Ledue TB, Haddow JE. Apolipoproteins and ischaemic heart disease: implications for screening. Lancet 1994;343:75-79.

30 Hecht HS, Superko R, Smith LK, McColgan BP. Relation of coronary artery calcium identified by electron beam tomography to serum lipoprotein levels and implications for treatment. Am J Cardiol 2001;87:406-412.

31 Grundy SM. Coronary calcium as a risk factor: role in global risk assessment: [Comment]. J Am Coll Cardiol 2001;37:1512-1515.

32 Janowitz, WR, Agatston AS, Viamonte M. Comparison of serial quantitative evaluation of calcified coronary artery plaque by ultrafast computed tomography in persons with and without obstructive coronary artery disease. Am J Cardiol 1991;68:1-6.

33 Maher JE, Bielak LF, Raz JA, Sheedy PF, Schwarz RS, Peyser PA. Progression of coronary artery calcification: a pilot study. Mayo Clin Proc 1999;74:347-355.

34 Budoff MJ, Lane KL, Bakhsheshi H, Mao S, Grassman BO, Friendman BC, Brundage BH. Rates of progression of coronary calcium by electron beam tomography. Am J Cardiol 2000;86:8-11.

35 Raggi P, Callister TQ, Lippolis NJ, Russo DJ. Cardiac events in patients with progression of coronary calcification on electron beam computed tomography (abstract). Radiology 1999;213:351.

36 Shah A, Sorochinsky B, Songshou M, Naik TK, Budoff MJ. Cardiac events and progression of coronary calcium score using electron beam tomography (abstract). Circulation 2000;102:II-604.

37 Calllister TQ, Raggi P, Cooil B, Lippolis NJ, Russo DJ. Effect of HMG-CoA reductase inhibitors on coronary artery disease as assessed by electron beam computed tomography. N Engl J Med 1998;339:1972-1978.

38 Achenbach S, Ropers D, Pohle K, Leber A, et al. Influence of lipid-lowering therapy on the progression of coronary artery calcification: a prospective evaluation. Circulation 2002;106:1077-1082.

39 Brown BG, Zhao X-Q, Chait A, Fisher LD, Cheung MC, Morse JS, Dowdy AA< Marino EK, et al. Simvastatin and niacin, antioxidant vitamins, or the combination for the prevention of coronary disease. N Engl J Med 2001;345:1582-1592.

40 Glagov S, Elliot W, Zarins CK, Stankunavicius R, Kolettis GJ. Compensatory enlargement of human atherosclerotic coronary arteries. N Engl J Med. 1987;316:1371-1375.

41 Grundy SM. Coronary plaque as a replacement for age as a risk factor in global risk assessment. Am J Cardiol 2001 Jul 19;88(2A):8E-11E.

42 Morin RL, Gerber TC, McCullough CH. Radiation dose in computed tomography of the heart. Circulation 2003;107:917-922.

43 Kondos GT, Hoff JA, Sevrukov A, et al. Electron beam tomography coronary artery calcium and cardiac events: a 37-month follow-up of 5635 initially asymptomatic low-to intermediate-risk adults. Circulation 2003;107:2571-2576.

44 Greenland P, Gaziano JM. Selecting asymptomatic patients for coronary computed tomography or electrocardiographic exercise testing. N Engl J Med 2003;349:465-73.

45 Stanford W, Thompson BH, Burns TL, Heery SD, Burr MC. Coronary artery calcium quantification at multi-detector row helical CT versus electron-beam CT. Radiology 2004;230:397-402.

46 Morin RL, Gerber TC, McCollough CH. Radiation dose in computed tomography of the heart. Circulation 2003; 107:917-922.

47 Waters D Craven TE, Lesperance J. Prognostic significance of progression of coronary atherosclerosis. Circulation 1993;87:1067-1075.

48 Azen SP. Mack WJ, Cashin-Hemphill L, et al. Progression of coronary artery disease predicts clinical coronary events. Circulation 1996;93:34-41.

49 Bruce Ra, Fisher LD, Hossack KF. Validation of exercise-enhanced risk assessment of coronary heart disease events: longitudinal changes in incidence in Seattle community practice. J Am Coll Cardiol 1985;5:875-881.

50 Multiple Risk Factor Intervention Trial Research Group. Exercise electrocardiogram and coronary heart disease mortality in the multiple risk factor intervention trial. Am J Cardiol 1985;55:16-24.

51 Mora S, Redberg RF, Cui Y, et al. Ability of exercise testing to predict cardiovascular and all-cause death in asymptomatic women: A 20-year follow-up of the Lipid Research Clinics Prevalence Study. JAMA 2003;290:1600-1607.

Appendix B
How to find a heart scanner
in your area

The availability of scanning devices with sufficient speed to image the coronary arteries has exploded over the last several years, putting a scanner within driving distance of nearly everyone in the U.S. At last count, there were nearly 100 EBT scanners in the U.S., all of which are listed below. MDCT devices are growing in number even more rapidly than EBT devices and will soon exceed the number of EBT scanners.

If a scanner that falls within an acceptable distance to your home is not listed, a call to major area hospitals sometimes will identify a scanning program on-site. Hospitals are just starting to show interest in these devices for heart scanning. Remember: before getting scanned, call and ask the center what kind of scanner they have. EBT and multi-detector scanners (sometimes called "multi-slice") are the preferred devices. The older spiral and helical (single detector) scanners are your last choice due to scanning imprecision and higher radiation exposure. Just as a car dealer can easily tell whether they're selling Fords or Chryslers, the scanning center staff should be able to tell you precisely what device is being used at their site. The brand or manufacturer is not an important issue. You may be told the device is a GE, Toshiba, Philips, or Siemens scanner, but the essential issue is whether or not it is an EBT or multidetector device and whether they have developed the local experience to permit coronary calcium scoring.

Scanner Locations

Alabama

University of Alabama at Birmingham
Kirklin Clinic
2000 6th Ave. South
Birmingham, AL 35249
Phone: 205–801–8606
GE LightSpeed Multi-detector scanner (4 slice)

Body Scan & Virtual Colonoscopy
350 Cypress Bend Drive
Gulf Shores, Alabama 36542
Phone: 251–967–7660 or Toll Free 866–656–7226
EBT scanner

Arizona

Arizona Heart Institute
2632 North 20th Street
Phoenix, AZ 85006
Phone: 602–212–1000
EBT scanner

John C. Lincoln Health Center
18404 North Tatum Blvd., Suite 103
Phoenix, Arizona 85032
Phone: 602–485–7482
GE LightSpeed Multi-detector scanner

BodyScan Imaging Center of Scottsdale
909 N. Scottsdale Rd.
Tempe, AZ 85281
Phone: 866–306–2639
EBT scanner

Southwest Preventive Imaging
4511 N. Campbell Ave., Suite 100
Tucson, AZ 85718
Phone: 520–529–4013
EBT scanner

California

Heart and Body Scan of America
5339 Truxton Ave.
Bakersfield, CA 92654
Phone: 661–863–0741
EBT scanner

Inner Vision Wellness Imaging
6185 Paseo Del Norte, Suite 110
Carlsbad, CA 92009
Phone: 760–804–9929
EBT scanner

Health Perfect Imaging
3070 Bristol St. Suite 190
Costa Mesa, CA 92626
Phone: 888–375–7226
EBT scanner

Heart Savers
Affiliated with Johns Hopkins Cardiology
20269 Stevens Creek Blvd.
Cupertino, CA 95014
Phone: 877–NEW–SCAN
EBT scanner

Full Body Scanning of Orange County
85 Fortune Drive, Suite 323
Irvine, CA 92618
Phone: 866–722–6872
Siemens multi-detector scanner (4 slice)

Heart Savers
Affiliated with Johns Hopkins Cardiology
4050 Barranca Pkwy, Suite 170
Irvine, CA 92604
Phone: 877–NEW–SCAN
EBT scanner

Lifeline Imaging—Laguna Hills
24012 Calle de La Plata
Laguna Hills, CA 92654
Phone: 866–432–7824
EBT scanner

Vital Imaging
9339 Genesee Avenue, Suite 150
San Diego, CA 92121
Phone: 858–713–9400 Toll-Free: 866–Vital–1–1 (866–848–2511)
EBT scanner

Cedars-Sinai Medical Center
8700 Beverly Blvd, Suite 1240
Los Angeles, CA 90048
Phone: 310–423–8000
EBT scanner

Heart Check Los Angeles
11859 Wilshire Blvd. Suite 110
Los Angeles, CA 90025
Phone: 800–NEW-TEST
EBT scanner

Advanced Body Scan of Newport
20311 Acacia Street, Suite 140
Newport Beach, CA 92660
Phone: 949–756–8200
EBT scanner

Vital Imaging
1120 W. La Veta, Suite 150
Orange, CA 92868
Phone: 714–547–1068 Toll-Free 866–Vital–1–1 (866–848–2511)
EBT scanner

Open System Imaging
44-215 Monterey Avenue
Palm Desert, CA 92260
Phone: 760–346–6413
Siemens Volume Zoom Multi-detector scanner (4 slice)

Vital Imaging
800 East Colorado Blvd., Suite 160
Pasadena, CA 91101
Phone: 626–585–0646 Toll-Free: 866–Vital–1–1 (866–848–2511)
EBT scanner

MD Imaging Incorporated
2020 Court St.
Redding, CA 96001
Phone: 530–243–1297
Multi-detector scanner (16-slice)

LifeScore
8899 University Center Lane, Suite 100
San Diego, CA 92122
Phone: 858–588–7267 Toll-Free: 877–543–3726
EBT scanner

Vital Imaging
Genesee Executive Plaza
9339 Genesee Avenue, Suite 150
San Diego, CA 92121
Phone: 866–Vital–1–1 (866–848–2511)
EBT scanner

Full Body Scanning of San Francisco
1825 Sacramento Street, Suite 100
San Francisco, CA 94109
Phone: 415–923–7474
GE LightSpeed scanner (8 slice)

Heartscan—San Franciso
389 Oyster Point Blvd.
South San Francisco, CA 94080
Phone: 650–872–7800
EBT scanner

Harbor-UCLA REI
St. Johns Cardiovascular Research Center Bldg.
1124 West Carson Street
Torrance, CA 90502
Phone: 310–222–2773
EBT scanner

HeartScan—Walnut Creek
2161 Ygnacio Valley road
Walnut Creek, CA 94598
Phone: 925–939–3003
EBT scanner

Colorado

Colorado Heart and Body Imaging
2490 W. 26th Avenue, Suite 110-A
Denver, CO 80211
Phone: 303–433–8800 Toll-Free: 800–800–3943
EBT scanner

Colorado Heart and Body Imaging
201 Columbine St.
Denver, CO 80206
Phone: 303–433–8800 Toll-Free: 800–800–3943
EBT scanner

Invision Imaging
499 E. Hampton Ave. Suite 170
Englewood, CO 80110
Phone: 303–788–4445
GE LightSpeed Multi-detector scanner (16 slice)

Connecticut

The Hospital of St. Raphael
1450 Chapel St.
New Haven, CT 06511
Phone: 203–789–3847
Multi-detector scanner

Delaware

Diagnostic Imaging Associates
Omega Imaging Associates
L-6 Omega Dr.
Newark, DE 19713
Phone: 302–738–9300
GE LightSpeed Multi-detector scanner

Florida

Body View
6000 Glade Rd. #1055
Boca Raton, FL 33431
Phone: 954–315–1600
Siemens Somatom Multi-detector scanner (16 slice)

Health Test Scan Center Boca Raton
301 Yamato Road, Suite 1240
Boca Raton, FL 33431
Phone: 561–241–9299
EBT scanner

Radiology Associates
Newporter Medical Mall
5539 Marine Pkwy. Suites 2,4,7 & 9
New Port Richey, Florida 34652
Phone: 727–815–3820
Siemens Volume Zoom Multi-detector scanner (4 slice)

Body Scan Imaging Center
3872 Oakwater Circle
Orlando, FL 32806
Phone: 407–851–9199
EBT scanner

Pembroke Pines Health Test Scan Center
700 N. Hiatus Rd., Ste. 105
Pembroke Pines, Fl., 33024
Phone: 877–432–7815
EBT scanner

Martin Memorial Health Services at
St. Lucie, FL
1095 NW St. Lucie, West Blvd.
Port St. Lucie, FL
Phone: 772–785–5566
GE LightSpeed Multi-detector scanner (16 slice)

Body Scan Imaging Center
3982 Bee Ridge Road, Bldg. H#A
Sarasota, FL 34233
Phone: 941–929–0148
EBT scanner

Martin Memorial Diagnostic Center
2396 SE Ocean Blvd.
Stuart, FL
Phone: 722–288–5817
GE LightSpeed Multi-detector scanner (16 slice)

Body Scan Imaging Center
3424 West Kennedy Boulevard
Tampa, FL 33609
Phone: 866–310–2639
EBT scanner

Georgia

Lifetest Imaging Center
Building I, Suite 9120
1140 Hammond Drive
Atlanta, GA 30328
Phone: 770–730–0119
EBT scanner

Hawaii

Kuakini Medical Center
347 North Kuakini Street.
Honolulu, Hawaii 96817
Phone: 808–547–9545
GE LightSpeed Multi-detector scanner (8 slice)

Holistica Hawaii
Hilton Hawaiian village
2005 Kalia Road
Honolulu, HI 96815
Phone: 808–951–6546
EBT scanner

Illinois

Heart Check America
University of Illinois Physicians Group
2010 South Arlington Heights Road, Suite 104
Arlington Heights IL 60005
Phone: 800–NEW–TEST
EBT scanner

BroMenn HeartCheck America
401 North Veterans Parkway
Bloomington, IL 61704
Phone: 309–268–3555
EBT scanner

Northwestern Memorial Hospital
251 East Huron Street
Chicago, IL 60611
Phone: 312–926–2000
EBT scanner

Rush Heart Scan
1725 West Harrison Avenue, Suite 025
Chicago, IL 60612
Phone: 800–SCAN–123
EBT scanner

University of Illinois Hospital
1740 W. Taylor Street Suite 2101
Chicago, IL 60612
Phone: 800–NEW–TEST
EBT scanner

Advanced Radiology Diagnostic Center
615 Valley View DR, Suite 101
Moline, IL
Phone: 309–743–0445
Siemens Multi-detector scanner (8-slice)

Edward Cardiovascular Institute
120 Spalding Drive, Suite 102
Naperville, IL 60540
Phone: 630–527–2802
EBT scanner

Scan America @ Prairie Heart Institute
619 East Mason
Springfield, IL 62701
Phone: 866–NOW–SCAN
EBT scanner

Iowa

Iowa Heart Center
411 Laurel Street, Suite A250
Des Moines, IA 50314
Phone: 515–235–5000
Siemens Volume Zoom Multi-detector scanner (4 slice)

University of Iowa Hospitals and Clinics
200 Hawkins Drive
Iowa City, Iowa 52242
Phone: 800–777–8442
EBT scanner

Indiana

Columbus Regional Hospital
2400 East 17th St.
Columbus, IN 47201
Phone: 812–379–4441 Toll-Free: 800–841–4938
Multi-detector scanner (4-slice)

Heart Check America
8333 Naab Road
Indianapolis, IN 46260
Phone: 800–NEW–TEST
EBT scanner

Unity Medical Center
1411 S. Creasy Lane, Suite 130
Lafayette, Indiana 47905
Phone: 765–447–7447
GE LightSpeed Multi-detector scanner (4 slice)

Rapid Scan
St. Joseph Regional Medical Center
801 East La Salle Ave.
South Bend, IN 46634
Phone: 219–280–5772
EBT scanner

Kansas

Body Scan Imaging Center
601 Westport Road
Kansas City, MO 64111
Phone: 866–931–2639
EBT scanner

Midwest EBT Cardiac Imaging
7521 West 119th
Overland, Park KS 66213
Phone: 913–469–5958
EBT scanner

Kentucky

Intecardia LifeCare Imaging
6420 Dutchmans Parkway, Suite 185
Louisville, KY 40205
Phone: 502–721–9898
EBT scanner

Owensboro Heart and Vascular
1200 Breckenridge Street, Suite 101
Owensboro, KY 42303
Phone: 270–683–8672
EBT scanner

Maryland

Virtual Physical
1838 Greene Tree Road, Suite 225
Pikesville, Maryland 21208-7115
Phone: 866–874–9742
Philips Multi-detector scanner

HeartSavers
Affiliated with Johns Hopkins Cardiology
110 W. Timonium Road Suite #1D
Timonium, MD 21093
Phone: 877–NEW–SCAN
EBT scanner

Massachusetts

Massachusetts General Hospital
40 Second Avenue, Suite 100
Waltham, MA 02451
Phone: 800–697–8296
GE LightSpeed Multi-detector (16 slice)

Weymouth MRI Diagnostic Imaging
420 Libbey Parkway
Weymouth, MA 02189
Phone:781–331–9880
Multi-detector scanner

Michigan

Early Warning Healthcare Institute
3100 Cross Creek Parkway, Suite 160
Auburn Hills, MI 48326
Phone: 248–371–9000
EBT scanner

Michigan Heart Imaging
G3239 Beecher Road
Flint, MI 48532
Phone: 810–733–6182
EBT scanner

EBT Heart and Body Imaging
26400 W. 12th Mile Road, Suite 114
Southfield, MI 48034
Phone: 248–358–3225
EBT scanner

Advanced Imaging of Michigan
2401 West Big Beaver Road, Suite 101
Troy, MI 48084
Phone: 248–816–9900
Siemens Multi-detector scanner (16-slice)

LifeScan Imaging of Michigan
11012 Thirteen Mile Rd.
Warren, MI
Phone: 517–669–1866
GE LightSpeed Multi-detector scanner

Minnesota

Minnesota Radiology Virtual Colonoscopy and Body Scan
4000 West 76th St.
Edina, MN 55435
Phone: 952–853–7226
Multi-detector scanner (16-slice)

HeartScan Minnesota
Minneapolis Heart Institute and Abbott
Northwestern Hospital Department of Radiology
800 East 28th Street
Minneapolis, MN 55407
Phone: 612–863–3500
EBT scanner

Minneapolis Radiology
2800 Campus Drive
Plymouth, MN 55441
Phone: 763–398–4400
Siemens Somatom Multi-detector scanner (4 Slice)

Mayo Clinic
Rochester Methodist Hospital
Charlton Building
Rochester, MN 55905
Phone: 507–284–2511
EBT scanner

Mississippi

Close to Biloxi, MS
Body Scan and Virtual Colonoscopy
350 Cypress Bend Dr.
Gulf Shores, AL 36542
Phone: 251–967–7660 or Toll Free 866–656–7226
EBT scanner

Missouri

Heart Check St. Louis
522 North New Ballas Road, Suite 113
Creve Coeur, MO 63141
Phone: 800–NEW–TEST
EBT scanner

BodyScan—Kansas City
601 Westport
Kansas City, MO 64111
Phone: 816–931–2639
EBT scanner

Town and Country
1176 Town and Country Common Drive
St Louis, MO 63017
Phone: 636–207–2210
Multi-detector scanner

Midwest Imaging and Prevention
605 Old Ballas Road, Suite 250
St. Louis, MO 63141
Phone: 314–997–3228
EBT scanner

Nebraska

Bryan LGH Medical Center
1600 S. 48th Street in Lincoln, NE
Phone: 402–481–8944
GE LightSpeed Multi-detector (16-slice)

LifeScan Preventative Imaging
2930 Pine Lake Road, Suite 111
Lincoln, NE 68516
Phone: 402–420–7999
EBT scanner

Nevada

Body Scan Imaging Center
2558 Wigwam Parkway
Henderson, NV 89074
Phone: 866–454–2639
EBT scanner

HeartScan-Las Vegas
2400 Tech Center Court
Las Vegas, NV 89128
Phone: 702–256–8282
EBT scanner

New Jersey

South Jersey Radiology Associates
1401 E. Route 70 Suite 9
Cherry Hill, NJ 08034
Phone: 856–428–4344
GE LightSpeed Multi-detector scanner (16 slice)

Hackensack University Medical Center
Preventive Cardiology Program
20 Prospect Avenue, Suite 200
Hackensack, NJ 07601
Phone: 201–996–3802
EBT scanner

Princeton Longevity Center
46 Vreeland Dr.
Skillman, NJ 08558
Phone: 609–430–0752
EBT scanner

Intecardia LifeCare Imaging
3 Sheila Drive
Tinton Falls, NJ 07724
Phone: 732–345–0900
EBT scanner

New York

Albany Advanced Imaging, P.L.L.C.
3 Atrium Drive
Albany, NY 12205
Phone: 518–438–0600
GE LightSpeed Multi-detector scanner (16-slice)

Sitron-Hammel Radiology Group P.C.
4277 Hempstead Tpke, Suite 200
Bethpage, NY 11714
Phone: 516–796–4340
GE LightSpeed Multi-detector scanner (4 slice)

Central Imaging
445 Kings Highway
Brooklyn, NY 11223
Phone: 866–886–7226
EBT scanner

Body Scan Imaging Center
301 E. 55th St
Manhattan NY, 10022
Phone: 212–829–1177
EBT scanner

Winthrop-University Hospital
259 First St.
Mineola, NY 11501
Phone: 866–WINTHROP
Phillips Multi-detector scanner (16-slice)

Inner Imaging
67 Irving Place
New York, NY 10003
Phone: 212–777–8900
EBT scanner

Body Scan Imaging Center
2975 Westchester Ave
Purchase, NY 10577
Phone: 914–697–9500
EBT Scanner

St. Francis Hospital
DeMatties Center for Research and Education
100 Port Washington Blvd.
Roslyn, NY 11576
Phone: 516–629–2000
EBT scanner

North Carolina

Cabarrus Radiologists
212 LePhillip Ct. NE, Suite 201
Concord, NC 28025
Phone: 704–786–0214
GE LightSpeed Multi-detector scanner (16 slice)

Raleigh Radiology
Blue Ridge
2605 Blue ridge Road, Suite 220
Raleigh, NC 27607
Phone: 919–784–3419
Phillips Multi-detector scanner (8 slice)

Ohio

HealthWise Center
5747 Perimeter Dr., Suite 105
Dublin, OH 43017
Phone: 614-652-5888
EBT scanner

Oklahoma

Integris Heart Hospital
3300 NW Expressway
Oklahoma City, OK 73112
Phone: 405–951–2277
Toll-Free: 888–951–2277
EBT scanner

Oregon

Heart Institute of the Cascades
2500 NE Neff Road
Bend, OR 97701-6015
Phone: 541–382–4321
EBT scanner

Open Advanced MRI and CT
9370 SW Greenburg Rd.
Grand Bldg., Suite J
Portland, OR 97223
Phone: 503–246–6666
GE LightSpeed Multi-detector scanner

Pennsylvania

Body Scan Imaging Center
2405 Easton Road
Willow Grove, PA 19090
Phone: 800–405–8851
EBT scanner

HeartCam Preventative Heart Care Center
3 Philadelphia Heart Institute Building
39th Street and Market
Philadelphia, PA 19104
Phone: 800–683–6942
EBT scanner

Pennsylvania Hospital
800 Spruce Street
Philadelphia, PA 19107
Phone: 215–829–3000 Toll-Free: 800–789–PENN
EBT scanner

Mercy Heart Institute
Department of Radiology
1400 Locust Street
Pittsburgh, PA 15219
Phone: 800–NEW–TEST
GE Multi-detector scanner

University of Pittsburgh Medical Center
Preventative Heart Care Center
120 Lytton Avenue, Suite 302
Pittsburgh, PA 15213
Phone: 412–683–5580
EBT scanner

South Carolina

Medical University of South Carolina
MUSC Heart & Vascular Center
169 Ashley Ave, PO Box 250341
Charleston, SC 29425
Phone: 843–792–1414 Toll-Free: 800–424–MUSC
Multi-detector scanner

South Carolina Heart Center
2001 Lauren St.
Columbia, SC 29204
Phone: 803–254–3278 Toll-Free: 800–714–3278
Siemens Multi-detector scanner

Charleston Clinic
234 Seven Farms road
Daniel Island, SC 29492
Phone: 843–576–3700
EBT scanner

Innervision
Patewood Business Center Bldg. 1
1 Marcus Drive
Greenville, SC 29615
Phone: 864–289–9977
EBT scanner

Tennessee

LifeTest Imaging Center
330 23rd Avenue North
Nashville, TN 37203
Phone: 615–321–5700
EBT scanner

Texas

Body Scan Imaging Center
3801 Cap of Tex Hwy North, #J210
Austin, TX 78746
Phone: 512–347–7226
EBT scanner

The Heart Hospital of Austin
HeartSavers CT
3801 N. Lamar Blvd.
Austin, TX 78756
Phone: 512–407–7283
EBT scanner

Cooper Clinic North
North Building
12200 Preston Road
Dallas, TX 75230
Phone: 972–560–2704
EBT Scanner

Cooper Clinic South
Department of Radiology
12200 Preston Road
Dallas, TX 75230
Phone: 972–239–7223
EBT scanner

University of Texas Southwest
5801 Forest Park
Rogers MRI Bldg.
Dallas, TX 75235
Phone: 214–648–5800
EBT scanner

Lifescan
2911 Oak Park Circle
Fort Worth, TX 76109
Phone: 800–905–SCAN
GE LightSpeed Multi-detector scanner

HeartScan—Houston
Scurlock Tower, Suite 610
6560 Fannin Street
Houston, TX 77030
Phone: 713–796–8940
EBT scanner

Houston Preventative Imaging
8800 Katy Freeway, Suite 105
Houston, TX 77024
Phone: 713–436–9090
EBT scanner

Vital Imaging-Houston
777 S. Post Oak Lane, Suite 100
Houston, TX 77056
Phone: 713–552–0045
EBT scanner

Colinas
349 Las Colinas Blvd., Suite C
Irving, TX 75039
Phone: 800–585–2702
EBT scanner

Covenant EBT
3615 19th Street
Lubbock, TX 79410
Phone: 806–725–2328
EBT scanner

ViaScan of Plano
3304 Communications Parkway, Suite 201
Plano, TX 75093
Phone: 972–403–1655
EBT scanner

Body Scan Imaging Center
2515 Babcock
San Antonio, TX 78229
Phone: 210–614–3158
EBT scanner

South Texas Radiology
7402 John Smith Drive
San Antonio, TX 78229
Phone: 210–614–4051
Siemens Multi-detector scanner (4 slice)

Utah

Accuscan Health Imaging
130 South 400 West
Salt Lake City, UT
Phone: 801–456–SCAN Toll-Free: 866–991–7226
GE LightSpeed Multi-detector scanner

Vital Imaging—Salt Lake City
3949 South 700 East, Suite 150
Salt Lake City, UT 84107
Phone: 866–VITAL–1–1
EBT scanner

HealthSouth Diagnostic Imaging
10011 Centennial Pkwy, #150
Sandy, UT 84070
Phone: 801–256–6400
Multi-detector scanner (16-slice)

Virginia

Intecardia LifeCare Imaging
7229 Forest Ave., Suite 108
Richmond, VA 23226
Phone: 804–285–SCAN
EBT scanner

HealthScreen Virginia
4668 Pembroke Blvd.
Virginia Beach, VA 23455-6423
Phone: 757–497–5433
Multi-detector scanner

Winchester Imaging
The Trex Center
160 Exeter Drive, Suite 104
Winchester, Virginia 22603
Phone: 540–545–4674
Siemens Multi-detector scanner (16-slice)

Washington

Vital Imaging Bellevue
1110 112th Ave. NE
Bellevue, WA 98004
Phone: 425–629–1015
EBT scanner

InHealth Imaging
20700 Bond Rd.
Paulsbo, WA 98370
Phone: 360-598-3141 Toll-Free: 888-837-8826
Multi-detector scanner

Life Screen Imaging
600 Broadway, Suite 170
Seattle, WA 98122
Phone: 206–292–7226
GE Ultra LightSpeed Multi-detector scanner

Swedish Heart Institute EBT Services
500 17th Ave.
Seattle, WA 98124
Phone: 206–320–4411
EBT scanner

Open Advanced MRI and CT
221-G NE 104th Ave., Suite 106
Vancouver, WA 98664
Phone: 360–253–2525
GE LightSpeed Multi-detector scanner

Washington, DC

Heart Check Washington DC
2401 Pennsylvania Avenue, N.W.
Washington, DC 20037
Phone: 202–467–0929
EBT scanner

Walter Reed Medical Center
Bldg. 2 Room 6Z39
Washington, DC 20307
Phone: 202–782–5111
EBT scanner

West Virginia

Greenbrier Clinic
320 West Main Street
White Sulphur Springs, WV 24986
Phone: 304–536–4870
EBT scanner

Wisconsin

Elmbrook Memorial Hospital
19333 W North Ave.
Brookfield, WI 53045
Phone: 262–780–4141
GE LightSpeed Multi-detector scanner (16-slice)

Sacred Heart Hospital
900 West Clairemont Avenue
Eau Claire, WI 54701
Phone: 715–839–4121
Multi-detector scanner

Milwaukee Heart Scan
10200 Innovation Drive, Suite 600
Milwaukee, WI 53226
Phone: 414–774–7600
EBT scanner

Wisconsin Heart Hospital
10,000 W. Bluemound Rd.
Wauwatosa, WI 53226
Phone: 414-778-7800
Philips 16-slice Multi-detector scanner

Example letter to insurance company to request reimbursement for heart scanning:

This is an example letter that your doctor can use to request insurance coverage for your EBT or multi-detector heart scan. Of course, you should change the names of the insured and specify the type of device used. You might also include any identifying numbers assigned to you by your insurance plan.

Re: *Mr. John Smith*
Member number: *1234–5678*

To whom it may concern:

I am writing on behalf of Mr. John Smith regarding payment for his CT heart scan performed at *Milwaukee Heart Scan.*

Heart scanning and calcium scoring are FDA-approved procedures. A recent American Heart Association and American College of Cardiology Consensus Panel stated that calcium scoring can be a useful tool to quantify sub-clinical coronary plaque.

The calcium score is the most powerful method available to identify asymptomatic people at risk for heart attack, superior to cholesterol values and stress testing (Wong et al, Am J Cardiol 2000;86:495–498). Early detection of asymptomatic coronary plaque can also reduce the need for expensive heart procedures. A high score identifies the need for intensive risk factor management in the hopes of substantially decreasing the likelihood of heart attack and bypass surgery. People at high-risk for coronary events can be identified early and appropriate preventive therapies instituted.

CT heart scanning and calcium scoring can also avoid unneeded heart catheterization. Persons with low calcium scores can often avoid this expensive procedure. (Raggi et al, American J. Cardiology 200; 85:283–288.)

In the case of *Mr. Smith*, his significant score has led to a program of vigorous prevention that I believe greatly minimizes *his/her* need for heart procedures. Although there is an upfront cost of the scan, the long-term financial savings are significant. *Mr. Smith's* score placed *him/her* in a very high-risk category for heart attack, despite *his* lack of symptoms.

I would therefore request your careful consideration in *Mr. Smith's* request for payment for these services.

Sincerely,

John Doe, M.D.

Appendix C
How to arrange lipoprotein testing in your area

The best place to start to obtain lipoprotein testing is with your own family physician, internist, or cardiologist. More and more doctors have at least heard about these tests. If your doctor is unable to provide this service, ask to be referred to another physician with expertise in lipoproteins. If your doctor is unaware of an expert in your area, refer to the listing below for helpful resources. The two testing laboratories listed can identify practitioners in your area who can both draw the blood sample and provide interpretation. Individual practicing physicians are not listed here, but the lipoprotein testing companies below can point you towards practitioners who may be able to assist you. As another option, ask the staff at the EBT or MDCT center you use whether lipoprotein testing is offered, also, since some centers have added blood drawing and physician interpretation of lipoproteins to their scanning services.

If your physician is willing to obtain the blood sample for you, the staff at the testing laboratories can help your physician and staff prepare the blood sample for testing. (The specimen needs to be prepared in a specific fashion and shipped on ice.) Alternatively, you can be directed to a "draw site" in your area for the blood sample to be drawn. These are general laboratories with staff who've received instruction on the proper procedure to follow. After the blood sample is obtained and submitted to either Liposcience or Berkeley HeartLabs, you will then need to see a physician for interpretation of these results. Once again, the two testing laboratories can steer you to knowledgeable physicians. You can also contact **Track Your Plaque** for interpretation (see below).

If you choose to see a physician identified by one of these testing labs, you should check with your health insurance carrier first to see whether you can see this practitioner within the restrictions of your health plan. Otherwise, you might be personally liable for part or all of the expenses incurred.

For physicians interested in learning more about lipoprotein analysis and its clinical application, the two resources listed below can point you in the right direction. Both LipoScience and Berkeley HeartLabs provide excellent educational materials and help professionals obtain the learning and experience necessary to begin applying these technologies.

The Liposcience website can be found at www.liposcience.com. You can e-mail the company to contact your local representative, who can then steer you towards physicians using the technology in your area. Or call 877–547–6837 and ask for your local representative for assistance.

The Berkeley HeartLab website can be found at www.berkeleyheartlab.com where you can find a "consumer hotline" (select the "In the news" button) to help identify practitioners using this lipoprotein testing technology in your area. You can also call 866–871–4408.

Once your blood has been drawn and the sample submitted to one of the laboratories above, results will be sent to the physician who ordered the test. If you would like interpretation through **Track Your Plaque**, forward the results to us by mail or fax and we will provide you with a physician interpretation of your results. The cost is $75 per consultation; a written interpretation will be sent to both you and the physician you designate. If you've had a coronary calcium score, this information would also be very helpful. Contact us at:

Track Your Plaque
William R. Davis, MD, FACC
2600 N. Mayfair Rd., Suite 950
Wauwatosa, WI 53226
Phone 414–456–1123
Fax 414–456–1766
Website: www.trackyourplaque.com

Example letter for response to insurance company for questions regarding lipoprotein testing:

(You can give a copy of this letter for your doctor to use. Be certain to choose either the NMR LipoProfile or the Berkeley HeartLab testing, since both are listed in the letter.)

July 23, 2004
Dear _____,

50% of patients who enter the emergency room experiencing a coronary event have "normal cholesterol". Standard cholesterol testing is simply *not* a good predictor of heart disease and coronary events. However, the results of a new, CLIA approved, diagnostic test called the *NMR LipoProfile/Berkeley HeartLab Gradient Gel Electropheresis* (choose one) now provides physicians with information to more effectively identify causes of heart disease. The *NMR LipoProfile/Berkeley HeartLab Gradient Gel Electropheresis* measures LDL particle number or apoprotein B, now considered the #1 predictor of heart disease progression from the Quebec Cardiovascular Study (Circulation-Lamarche et al, 1997; 95:69–75) and Cardiovascular Health Study (Kuller et al AHA November 2001).

Furthermore, the *NMR LipoProfile/Berkeley HeartLab Gradient Gel Electropheresis* measures LDL and HDL lipoprotein subclass levels and size and provides a risk assessment panel in addition to conventional lipid values.

Currently, my patients with ___*(insurer name)*_____are not covered for the *NMR LipoProfile/Berkeley HeartLab Gradient Gel Electropheresis* test. The *NMR LipoProfile/Berkeley HeartLab Gradient Gel Electropheresis* test is a medical necessity for my patients.

In order to obtain the medical data I need to determine my patients cardiovascular risk and treatment path, without the *NMR LipoProfile,/Berkeley HeartLab Gradient Gel Electropheresis* I would have to order four tests: standard cholesterol panel $80, direct LDL-C $80, apoB-100 $80, apoA-1 $65, which would total over $300 to the insurance company, and for inferior information.

The *NMR LipoProfile/Berkeley HeartLab Gradient Gel Electropheresis* test allows me to better prevent heart disease, design more effective treatments and allow early identification of risk, because it provides me with six times the information that a standard cholesterol test does.

Please place the *NMR LipoProfile/Berkeley HeartLab Gradient Gel Electropheresis* on the___*(insurer name)*_____ formulary to ensure complete coverage for my patients. Please contact me and I would be happy to address any questions that you might have.

Sincerely,
John Smith, M.D.

Appendix D
Resources to help you find tools and products used in Track Your Plaque

l-arginine powders and products

L-arginine can be found in most health food stores as 500–1000 mg capsules. However, because of the dose used in **Track Your Plaque** of 3000–6000 mg twice a day, it's a lot easier to use a powder preparation. (Taking 500 mg capsules to achieve a dose of 6000 mg twice a day would mean taking 24 capsules a day!). Powdered l-arginine is a bit more difficult to locate. Some sources are listed below.

Sourcenaturals.com

This website lists retailers that sell the SourceNaturals brand of l-arginine powder.

The Life Extension Foundation

The Life Extension Foundation is an excellent source of information and scientific reviews of new and unusual health ideas. (Despite its name, this organization has a lot of information beyond "life extension".) The products they sell are high-quality. There's a $75 per year membership fee, though it does entitle you to reduced pricing on various supplements. They are distributors of the PowerMaker brand of l-arginine powder, the form that we've used for several years in our patients (around $35 per canister, which lasts about 4–8 weeks, depending on dose).

> Life Extension Foundation
> P.O. Box 229120
> Hollywood, FL 33022
> Phone 800–544–4440
> Website: www.lef.org

If you're looking for variety, the *Heart Bar* products are food bars that contain "therapeutic" doses of l-arginine (6000 mg per bar). They also have an excellent l-arginine powder. These are among the best products you will find as sources for l-arginine, though they are quite expensive. The bars also contain vitamins C and E; vitamins B6, B12, and folate to lower homocysteine, and soy protein. The recently improved bars actually taste pretty good. The website contains helpful background information, including some of the scientific data on l-arginine use to prevent coronary disease. The focus of much of the Heart Bar product literature is the reduction of angina (chest pain) for people with established symptomatic coronary disease and reduction of claudication, or cramping in the calf muscles while walking due to atherosclerosis in the leg arteries. But l-arginine products are just as useful—perhaps even more so—when taken earlier in the plaque growth process, when there is "silent" plaque. The company seems to be pushing customers into a multi-level marketing program in which you both buy and sell products. However, you can choose, of course, to just buy enough for personal use.

> Cooke Pharma, Inc.
> Phone: 888–808–6838
> Website: www.heartbar.net

Fish oil

Standard fish oil preparations are available from just about any health food store or grocery store. However, for those of you who are simple unable to tolerate the fishy odor or aftertaste, a fabulous non-fishy alternative is available from the Pharmax company. Their Frutol product is a fruit-flavored puree that has no fishy taste whatsoever, and is very reasonably priced.

> Pharmax LLC
> Phone: 425-467-8054
> Website: www.pharmaxllc.com

Calorie counting pedometers

Calorie counting pedometers are widely available. You can find them in sporting goods stores and in sporting goods departments of major retail stores. Many health clubs carry a selection, also. Try to choose a pedometer that can provide both *calories* expended as well as *number of steps* taken, since both can be helpful perspectives on physical activity. There are several excellent devices that are reliable and inexpensive (around $20). Omron, Acumen, and Digi-Walker brands have worked well in our experience. Acumen also has a water-proof device that you can use for swimming.

In addition to retail stores, there are numerous websites that distribute calorie counters. Enter either "calorie counter" or one of the brand names into your search engine. Or you can try one of these sites:

www.bodytrends.com

www.acumeninc.com

Soy protein and other soy products

Proponents of soy have amassed a huge amount of helpful literature for the uninitiated. These organizations and websites have well-prepared and well-researched background information, recipes, and advice on how to choose products.

United Soybean Board

424 Second Ave. West

Seattle, WA 98119

Phone: 800–825–5769

website: www.soyfoods.com

I particularly recommend the Soybean Board's website which is well-designed and full of useful information. An alternative website maintained by the United Soybean Board can be found at www.talksoy.com. This website is a concise source for new developments in soy products and science.

Soyfoods Association of North America

1723 U Street, NW

Washington, DC 20009

Phone 202–986–5600

Website: www.soyfoods.org

Another helpful website full of information, recipes, as well as updates on new scientific developments on soy-related issues.

Genisoy Products Company

2351 N. Watney Way, Suite C

Fairfield, CA 94533

Phone: 888–436–4769

Website: www.genisoy.com.

Genisoy is a company selling soy products but is nonetheless an excellent source of information.

> DuPont Protein Technologies
> Marketing Communications, 5C
> P.O. Box 88940
> St. Louis, MO 63188
> Phone: 800–325–7108
> Website: solae.com

If you're looking for a good overview of soy, the solae.com site is concise and easy to navigate.

Progesterone and testosterone creams

Natural human progesterone can be administered as a topical cream or taken orally in pill form. Testosterone can be taken topically as a cream or as patches. Both progesterone in pill form and testosterone in patch form are available at most pharmacies by prescription. Patients especially like cream forms, however, as they disappear from site on application, are nearly odorless, and are generally much less expensive than other prescription forms. (Many insurers will not cover hormonal preparations.)

If you're interested in using a cream preparation, you will need to have a special pharmacy called a "compounding" pharmacy make up your cream. Unlike regular pharmacies, compounding pharmacies can specially prepare prescriptions to your doctor's specifications. The pharmacist can be helpful in compounding human progesterone or testosterone in a cream base that you apply to your chest or arms for absorption. Estrogen and DHEA creams are also available by prescription. An excellent compounding pharmacy is The Women's International Pharmacy in Madison, Wisconsin and Sun City West, Arizona. (Despite the name, they formulate all kinds of hormonal preparations for both men and women.) The Women's International Pharmacy provides first-class service and will send you loads of information when you fill your prescription. They accept prescriptions from your doctor by FAX or by mail.

> Women's International Pharmacy
> 5708 Monona Drive
> Madison, WI 53716
> Phone 608–221–7800
> FAX 608–221–7819

13925 W. Meeker Blvd, Suite 13
Sun City West, AZ 85375
Phone 623–214–7700
FAX 623–214–7708
Also: Toll free phone 800–279–5708, FAX 800–279–8011
Website: www.wipws.com, e-mail info@wipws.com

You can also consult the phone book under "pharmacies". Compounding pharmacies will often advertise the fact that they can compound prescriptions.

Index

A

Achenbach, MD, Stephan, 196, 203, 206, 208
Adult Treatment Panel III, 44
   LDL cholesterol and, 80, 87, 92-93, 95, 112-113, 119, 121-122, 134, 140, 162-163, 176
Agatston score, 60, 196
Agatston, MD, Arthur, 60
Alcohol, 24, 132-133, 151, 190
Almonds, 88, 97-98, 101, 115, 120, 134, 165-166, 171, 174, 176, 179
   LDL cholesterol and, 80, 87, 92-93, 95, 112-113, 119, 121-122, 134, 140, 162-163, 176
   lipoprotein (a) and, 97,98,165
American Heart Association, 18, 20, 36, 235
   diet, 1, 5, 13-17, 24-25, 71, 73, 80, 89, 93, 101-102, 108-112, 114-119, 121, 125-128,
     130-132, 135, 139, 143-145, 148-149, 152-153, 155, 158, 166, 170, 176, 178, 180-181,
     183, 190
   policy statement on stress testing, 36
Ankle-brachial index, 53-54
Anti-oxidants, 167, 170
Apoprotein B, 90-94, 97, 102-103, 105-106, 112, 119-120, 122, 140, 153, 162, 166, 171,
     175, 239, *See* LDL particle number
Arad, MD, Yadon, 206
Atkins diet, 110, 152-153
Atorvastatin, 83-84, 91
Austin, Dr. Melissa, 6

B

Beans, 88, 119-120, 129-130
   LDL cholesterol and, 80, 87, 92-93, 95, 112-113, 119, 121-122, 134, 140, 162-163, 176
Benecol, 88, 162, 171
   LDL cholesterol and, 80, 87, 92-93, 95, 112-113, 119, 121-122, 134, 140, 162-163, 176
Berkeley HeartLabs, 83, 105, 187, 237
Beta-carotene, 167, 170
Bioimpedance, 144, 146
Bitter orange, 148

Blood pressure, 12, 19, 29, 43, 53-54, 72, 81, 89, 97-98, 112, 114, 118, 121, 125, 133-135,
    140, 147, 160, 162, 167-168, 184
  coenzyme Q10 and, 98
  exercise effects on, 141
Body fat, 144, 146-147, 150
Body fat percent, 144, 146
Body mass index, 144
Bodytrends, 243
Boyd, PhD, Douglas, 5, 49
Brown, MD, Greg, 167
Budoff, MD, Matt, 205-207
Bypass surgery, 2, 12, 16, 18-23, 25, 30, 32, 47, 54, 56, 62, 64, 67-68, 78-79, 88, 176, 181-182,
    188, 235

C

Caffeine, 24, 132-133, 141, 148
Calcium, 4, 6, 8, 15, 19, 29-30, 32, 35, 46, 48-51, 56, 58-65, 67-69, 71, 73, 78, 81, 100,
    148, 155-157, 164, 178, 182, 186, 193-209, 235, 238
  and atherosclerotic plaque, 50, 194
  coronary, 2-16, 18-33, 35-37, 39, 43-58, 60, 62-70, 72-73, 77-80, 82, 84, 87, 90, 92-94,
      99-102, 104, 107, 109-112, 114, 126, 135, 137-139, 143, 147-148, 153, 155, 157-
      162, 166-168, 174, 176-178, 180-182, 185-186, 189-191, 193-209, 235, 238-239, 242
Calcium pyruvate, 148, 155-156
Calcium score, 15, 46, 51, 56, 58-64, 67, 69, 78, 100, 157, 178, 182, 186, 193, 196-204,
    207, 235, 238
  "red flags", 61
  Agatston, 60, 195-196, 205-207
  bypass surgery and, 176
  catheterization and, 9
  diabetes and, 78, 127, 135, 139
  heart attack risk and, 59-61
  metabolic syndrome and, 139
  percentile rank, 59-61, 67, 195, 199, 201, 204
  reduction of, 71, 110, 164, 203, 242
  risk of heart attack with increasing scores, 66, 73
  stents and, 19
  stress testing and, 61, 200
Calcium scoring, 4, 6, 30, 49, 51, 61-62, 65, 68, 73, 78, 193, 196-198, 200-204, 206, 209, 235
  methods, 3, 7-8, 17, 23-24, 29, 39, 51, 67, 71, 82-83, 103, 131, 147, 162, 165, 170, 187,
      195-196
  volumetric, 196, 206

Callister, MD, Traci, 6
calcium scoring volumetric, 196, 208
Calorie expenditure, 153-155
Cannon, MD, Christopher, 83
Carotid, 18, 52-53, 159, 167
  intimal-medial thickness, 52-53
  ultrasound, 7, 29, 36-38, 47-48, 52-53, 159
Catheterization, 2, 5, 9, 18-20, 23-25, 31, 37-38, 47-48, 50-51, 62-64, 177, 235
Cerivastatin, 203-204
Cholesterol, 4, 12-13, 25-26, 29, 33, 43-47, 52, 54, 57, 71, 77-84, 87-89, 91-95, 97-98,
    100-109, 112-113, 115, 119-122, 126, 134, 140, 162-166, 168-169, 171-183, 185, 187,
    201, 203-204, 235, 239
  failure to identify silent heart disease, 2, 43-45, 77-80
  National Cholesterol Education Program, 12, 44
Cholesterol, total, 91
Coenzyme Q10, 98, 168, 174
  blood pressure and, 12, 112, 125, 134-135, 147, 160
  lipoprotein (a) and, 98
  muscle aches and, 168-169
Conjugated linolenic acid, 152
Cooke Pharma, 161, 242
Cooper Aerobics Center, 140
Corn syrup, 90, 122-123, 126, 131, 134
  high-fructose, 90, 122, 126, 131
Coronary, 2-16, 18-33, 35-37, 39, 43-58, 60, 62-70, 72-73, 77-80, 82, 84, 87, 90, 92-94,
    99-102, 104, 107, 109-112, 114, 126, 135, 137-139, 143, 147-148, 153, 155, 157-162,
    166-168, 174, 176-178, 180-182, 185-186, 189-191, 193-209, 235, 238-239, 242
  arteries—anatomy, 28
  artery—remodeling, 31, 36, 37, 197
  bypass surgery, 2, 12, 16, 18-23, 25, 30, 32, 47, 54, 56, 62, 64, 67-68, 78-79, 88, 176,
    181-182, 188, 235
  calcium, 4, 6, 8, 15, 19, 29-30, 32, 35, 46, 48-51, 56, 58-65, 67-69, 71, 73, 78, 81, 100,
    148, 155-157, 164, 178, 182, 186, 193-209, 235, 238
  calcium score, 15, 46, 51, 56, 58-64, 67, 69, 78, 100, 157, 178, 182, 186, 193, 196-204,
    207, 235, 238
  calcium score
  calcium score Agatston, 60, 195-196
  calcium score and CRP, 112
  calcium score and events, 60-61, 66, 198-200
  calcium score and heart attack prediction, 60-61, 66, 198-200

calcium score and rate of increase, 66-67, 70, 202-203
calcium score and severity of blockage, 59, 196-198
calcium score and stenosis severity, 59, 196-198
calcium score and stress testing, 36-39, 61, 63, 64, 137, 196-198, 200
calcium score percentile rank, 201
calcium score reproducibility, 195-196
calcium score, reduction of, 70-73, 203-204
calcium scoring, 4, 6, 30, 49, 51, 61-62, 65, 68, 73, 78, 193, 196-198, 200-204, 206, 209, 235
calcium scoring, volumetric, 196
plaque, 17, 19-39, 41, 43-73, 75, 77-85, 87-104, 106-112, 114, 116, 118, 120-124, 126-128, 130-132, 134-144, 146-148, 150, 152-162, 164, 166-168, 170, 172-191, 193-198, 200-208, 210, 212, 214, 216, 218, 220, 222, 224, 226, 228, 230, 232, 234-235, 237-238, 240-242, 244, 248, 250, 252, 254, 256, 258
plaque as risk factor, 37-39, 45-47
plaque burden, 38, 194-195, 197, 204
plaque composition, 29, 49
plaque detection, 5-6, 55, 200
plaque detection, history of, 5-6
plaque measurement, 8, 46, 55
plaque measurement, MRI, 30, 54-55
plaque regression, 19, 23, 73, 81
plaque rupture, 8, 59, 158
plaque, causes, 80-82
plaque, minor, 8
plaque, silent, 3, 5, 7, 37, 51
remodeling, 31, 36-37, 197
risk of heart attack, 3, 5, 44, 46-47, 61, 66, 73, 78, 100-101, 115, 121, 139, 167-168
stents, 7, 16, 19, 32, 46-47, 64, 67, 79, 181
ultrasound, 7, 29, 36-38, 47-48, 52-53, 159
Coronary artery disease, 27, 78, 80, 193, 205-208
development of, 63, 72, 80, 120, 194, 202, 205
in children, 30
likelihood of, 12, 32, 44-46, 57-59, 63, 70-71, 88, 93, 98, 122-123, 179, 182, 197-198, 235
medical therapy, 19
procedural treatment of, 20-23
silent, 8, 25, 36-37, 39, 51, 54, 57, 185, 190, 206, 242
symptoms, 1-4, 7-11, 14-15, 30, 33, 36-39, 46, 53, 62-64, 73, 79-80, 84, 125, 150, 175-179, 181-182, 193-194, 198, 202, 204, 235

symptoms of, in women, 14
  unstable symptoms, 15, 79, 176, 179
Coronary Artery Surgery Study, 46
Coronary bypass, 2, 16, 18, 20-21, 26, 177
  cost of, 18, 68, 83, 104, 235
  hospital revenues and, 20-21
  hospitals and, 18, 52, 218
C-reactive protein, 81, 104-106, *See* inflammation
  calcium score and, 15, 199, 204
  small LDL and, 96, 109, 111, 115, 122, 126-127, 147, 153, 173
  treatment of, 13, 78, 87, 96-97, 99-100, 106, 151, 175
Crohn's disease, 157, 161, 164
Curcumin, 165

D

DHEA, 151-152, 155-156, 170, 244
Diabetes, 12, 57, 72, 78, 89-90, 105, 120, 122-128, 135, 139, 166, 200
Diet, 1, 5, 13-17, 24-25, 71, 73, 80, 89, 93, 101-102, 108-112, 114-119, 121, 125-128, 130-132, 135, 139, 143-145, 148-149, 152-153, 155, 158, 166, 170, 176, 178, 180-181, 183, 190
  Atkins, 110, 152-153
  carbohydrate restriction, 102, 127, 152
  low-fat, 5, 13, 24-25, 89-90, 108-112, 116, 118, 123, 126-127, 130, 134-135, 152, 180
  South Beach, 152
  Sugar Busters, 152
  weight loss, 110, 117-118, 152-153, 155
  Zone, 108, 152
DuPont Protein Technologies, 244

E

Electron-beam tomography, 8, 49, 55, 194, *See* Heart scan
  development of., 63, 72, 80, 120, 194, 202, 205, *See* Ultra-fast CT
  radiation exposure, 65, 209
  scanner locations, 210
Electropheresis, 82-83, 96, 105-106, 175, 239-240, *See* Berkeley HeartLabs
Ephedra, 148
European Concerted Action on Thrombosis and Disabilities Angina Pectoris Study, 101
Exercise, 12-14, 22, 24, 26, 33, 36, 43, 71, 73, 89, 94, 97, 101, 109-110, 117, 124, 132, 136-149, 151, 155, 157, 169, 175, 179, 187-190, 207-208
  blood pressure effects, 53

blood sugar, effects on, 141
    goals, 103, 106-107, 139-140, 143, 154, 175, 183, 187
    HDL effects on, 89, 140
    LDL particle size, effects on, 94, 141
    lipid and lipoprotein effects of, 140
    triglycerides, effects on, 141
    weight control, 118, 140, 151
Ezetimibe, 88, 101
    C-reactive protein and, 176, 178
    LDL cholesterol and, 80, 87, 92-93, 95, 112-113, 119, 121-122, 134, 140, 162-163, 176

F

Familial hypertriglyceridemia, 90
Fat, 1, 14, 24, 32-33, 35, 81-82, 88, 97, 102, 108-119, 125, 130, 133, 135, 143-144, 146-148, 150-153, 157, 166, 181, 183
    counting grams, 116-118
    hydrogenated, 88, 93, 102, 111-113, 116-117, 122, 125, 135
    monounsaturated, 89, 115-118, 127, 134-135, 163, 166, 181
    polyunsaturated, 113-117
    saturated, 1, 88, 93, 102, 110-113, 115-117, 119, 130, 135, 152-153, 158
Fiber, 88, 101, 110, 118-122, 125, 128-130, 134-135, 163, 165-166, 188
    counting grams, 119
    soluble vs. insoluble, 118-120
Fibrinogen, 81-82, 101-102, 105, 115, 158, 173, 176
    fenofibrate and, 102
    fish oil and, 95, 97, 102, 183
    niacin and, 102
    treatment of, 13, 78, 87, 96-97, 99-100, 106, 151, 175
Fish oil, 81-82, 89-90, 95-98, 101-103, 114-115, 157-159, 171, 173, 176, 178, 180, 182-183, 242, See Omega-3 fatty acids
    available preparations, 157-159, 242
    effects of, 3, 16, 80, 88, 94, 99, 102-103, 118, 125, 132, 140, 143, 145, 149, 151, 158, 167, 170
    intolerance, 89, 105, 139, 159, 166
    lipoprotein(a) and, 98, 115
    sources of, 88, 115, 118-119, 121, 134, 188
    VLDL and, 83, 90, 102, 104, 122, 126, 145
    where to obtain, 242
Flavonoids, 110, 121, 134, 165, 167, 170
Flaxseed, 90, 97-98, 114-115, 118, 120, 122, 126, 131, 158, 162-165, 171, 176, 179
    lipoprotein(a) and, 97, 98, 115

Flaxseed oil, 90, 114 115, 158, 164, *See* Omega-3 fatty acids
Food, 88, 95, 109, 113, 115, 119-123, 125, 127-128, 130-133, 135-136, 144, 154, 166, 169,
    180, 183, 241-242
  habits, 6, 14, 17, 108-109, 124, 130, 132, 135, 138-139, 141, 145, 183, 189-190
  unprocessed, 120-125, 129, 135, 183
Framingham Trial, 45

G

Garlic, 133-134, 165
Genisoy Products Co., 243-244
Glycemic index, 89, 122-131, 134-135, 163, 166
  food choices and, 125-129
  lipoprotein effects of, 140
  table, 56-57, 60, 118, 123, 126, 190, 198
Grape seed extract, 170
Green tea catechin, 165
Guarana, 148
Gugulipid, 88
  LDL cholesterol and, 80, 87, 92-93, 95, 112-113, 119, 121-122, 134, 140, 162-163, 176

H

HATS Trial, 167
HDL cholesterol, 25, 87, 89, 92, 102-103, 106, 109, 113, 126, 140, 173-180, 182-183,
    187, 201
  exercise and, 12-13, 24, 109, 136-138, 140, 144-145, 148, 157, 169, 179, 189
  exercise effects on, 89, 140, 144
  fish oil and, 95, 97, 102, 183
  low-fat diet and, 89, 108-109
  weight and, 93-94, 109, 135, 144-145
HDL subclasses, 95
Heart attack, 1, 3-23, 25-28, 30-33, 36-39, 43-48, 51-54, 56-61, 63, 66, 68-71, 73, 77-81,
    84, 88, 92-93, 98-101, 114-115, 121, 132-133, 137-140, 144, 148, 158-159, 163, 167-168,
    173, 175-177, 179-180, 182, 186, 189, 191, 235
  as failure of prevention, 8, 23
  mild plaques and, 32, 37-39, 45-47
  plaque rupture and, 8, 32, 59
Heart disease, 27, 30, 33, 36, 39, 43-45, 47, 49, 51-57, 60, 62-68, 77-79, 82, 84, 87-90,
    92-93, 95-97, 99, 109-111, 118, 121, 131, 133, 135, 138-139, 147, 172-173, 175-177,
    180-181, 185-186, 189-191, 202, 207-208, 239
  silent, 8, 25, 36-37, 39, 51, 54, 57, 185, 190, 206, 242

Heart rate, 142-143, 145, 147, 202
  exercise goals, 142-143
Heart scan, 2, 8, 13, 15, 25, 46, 51, 56-62, 65-68, 70-73, 77-80, 83-84, 88, 92, 97-98,
    104-106, 111-112, 136, 138-140, 147, 173-174, 176-180, 182, 184-188, 217, 234-235,
    See Coronary calcium
  bypass surgery and, 176
  catheterization and, 9
  cost, 18, 37, 45, 55, 68, 83, 104, 146, 153, 159, 200, 235, 238
  development of, 63, 72, 80, 120, 194, 202, 205
  heart attack risk and, 60-61, 66, 198-200
  insurance coverage, 68, 235
  scanner locations, 210
  severity of blockage and, 59, 196-198
  stents and, 19
  stress testing and, 61, 200
  technologies, 3-5, 17, 23, 30, 55, 62, 64-65, 69, 182, 202, 238, 244
Hecht, MD, Harvey, 201
High fructose corn syrup, 123, 126, 131, 134
Hodis, MD, Howard, 52
Hoff, PhD, Julie, 206, 208
Homocysteine, 83, 99, 104-107, 141, 175-176, 178-179, 181, 242
  treatment of, 13, 78, 87, 96-97, 99-100, 106, 151, 175
Hydrogenated fat, 102, 112-113
Hydroxycitric acid, 152
Hyperphagia, 126

I

IDL, 96, *See* Intermediate-density lipoprotein
Inflammation, 7, 72, 81, 100, 168, 178, *See* c-reactive protein
  plaque, 17, 19-39, 41, 43-73, 75, 77-85, 87-104, 106-112, 114, 116, 118, 120-124, 126-
    128, 130-132, 134-144, 146-148, 150, 152-162, 164, 166-168, 170, 172-191, 193-
    198, 200-208, 210, 212, 214, 216, 218, 220, 222, 224, 226, 228, 230, 232, 234-235,
    237-238, 240-242, 244, 248, 250, 252, 254, 256, 258
Inositol hexaniacinate, 170, *See* No-flush niacin
Insulin, 105, 117, 121, 123-124, 126-127, 139, 141, 143, 152
  and glycemic index, 126-127
  sensitivity, 19, 100, 124, 127, 141, 153, 197-198
Intermediate-density lipoprotein, 96-97
Isoflavones, 164

K

Kondos, MD, George, 60
Krauss, Dr. Ronald, 6, 83
Krauss, MD, Ronald, 117-118

L

L-arginine, 97, 134, 156, 159-162, 166-167, 170, 173, 176, 178, 180, 182-183, 241-242
    preparations, 95, 98, 148-149, 158, 161-163, 168-170, 242, 244
    side-effects, 45, 95, 98, 148, 150, 152, 169
    where to obtain, 241-242
L-carnitine, 97-98, 152, 171, 177
    lipoprotein(a) and, 97, 98
LDL cholesterol, 1, 12, 33, 43-46, 57, 78, 80, 82-84, 87-88, 92-95, 97-98, 100-103, 105-106,
    108, 112-113, 119, 121-122, 134, 140, 162-166, 168-169, 171-181, 183, 187, 201,
    203-204
    Adult Treatment Panel III and, 44
    almonds and, 88, 101, 115, 171, 176, 179
    beans and, 130
    Benecol and, 88, 162
    ezetimibe and, 88
    flaxseed and, 97, 164-165
    gugulipid and, 88
    heart attack and, 5-6, 11, 13, 15, 17, 25, 38, 44, 46, 68-71, 99-100, 139, 235
    Metamucil and, 88, 164
    National Health and Nutritional Survey and, 44
    NCEP guidelines and, 12
    nutritional adjuncts to lower, 162-166
    nuts and, 89, 118, 126, 134, 138, 181
    oat bran and, 95, 127, 165, 174
    pantetheine and, 88
    pectin and, 88, 119, 120
    phytosterols and, 164, 166
    policosanol and, 88, 169
    psyllium seed and, 165
    red yeast and, 88, 169
    soy protein powder and, 88
    statin agents and, 88, 93
    Take Control and, 88
    treatment goals, 175

vitamin C and, 166, 167, 170

walnuts and, 120, 166

Zetia and, 88

LDL particle number, 90-94, 96-97, 102-107, 112, 119-120, 122, 140, 147, 153, 162, 171, 173-179, 181, 183, 239, *See* apoprotein B

reduction of, 71, 110, 164, 203, 242

statin agents and, 93

LDL, small, 83, 89-90, 93-98, 100, 102-103, 106, 109, 111, 115, 122, 124, 126-127, 144-145, 147, 153, 163, 165, 171, 173-181, 183

Life Extension Foundation, 241

Lifestyle Heart Trial, 24-25, *See* Ornish, MD, Dean

Linolenic acid, 114, 152, 158, 163, 166

Lipids, 67, 82-84, 102-104, 107, 111, 140, 143, 155, 179, 185-188

lipoproteins vs., 82-84

Lipitor, 83, 91, 93

Lipoic acid, 170

Lipoprotein, 4, 6, 14, 16, 66-67, 71, 73, 78-80, 82-84, 87, 89-93, 96-98, 101-107, 109-112, 114-115, 117-118, 122, 125, 127, 135-141, 143-145, 147, 155, 157-160, 165, 170, 173-181, 183, 186-188, 207, 237-239

analysis, 4, 73, 78-79, 93, 102-103, 109, 159, 174, 177-180, 186-188, 195-197, 199, 201, 237

testing, how to obtain, 237-238

Lipoprotein (a), 97-98

almonds and, 88, 101, 115, 171, 176, 179

blood pressure and, 12, 112, 125, 134-135, 147, 160

Coenzyme Q10 and, 98

estrogens and, 98

fish oil and, 95, 97, 102, 183

flaxseed and, 97, 164-165

l-carnitine and, 97, 98

niacin and, 97, 98

nutritional treatments, 97, 98

testosterone and, 150

treatment of, 13, 78, 87, 96-97, 99-100, 106, 151, 175

Lipoproteins, 4, 6, 23, 67, 71, 73, 80-84, 87, 89, 92, 96, 102-103, 105-106, 109, 111, 126, 135, 140, 143, 153, 155, 175, 183, 185-188, 237, *See* LipoScience, *See* Berkeley HeartLabs, *See* NMR, electropheresis

Berkeley HeartLabs, 83, 105, 187, 237

development of, 63, 72, 80, 120, 194, 202, 205

electropheresis, *See* Berkeley HeartLabs

exercise effects on, 140-141
fish oil, effects on, 157-159
lipids vs., 82-84
measurement, 4, 6, 8, 14, 23, 30, 46, 53, 55, 66, 81, 195
NMR, 6, 82-83, 92, 96-97, 104-106, 173, 175, 178, 180, 239-240
nuclear magnetic resonance of, 6, 83
suggested panels, 104-105
treatment goals, 175
vs. lipids, 82-84
LipoScience, 83, 104-105, 186-187, 237-238
Low-fat diet, 13, 24-25, 89, 111, 118
Ornish, 24-25, 108

M

Ma huang, 148
Magnetic resonance imaging, 6, 30, 54
Malabsorption, 161, 164
McCully, MD, Kilmer, 99
Metabolic syndrome, 72, 89, 97, 105, 127, 139, 147, 153
Metamucil, 88, 101, 164, 171
LDL cholesterol and, 80, 87, 92-93, 95, 112-113, 119, 121-122, 134, 140, 162-163, 176
Monounsaturated fatty acids, 89, 115-116, 118, 135
Multi-detector scanners, 64, 209, *See* heart scan
radiation exposure, 65, 209
scanner locations, 210
Multiple Risk factor Intervention Trial, 44, 208

N

National Cancer Institute nutritional approach, 131
National Cholesterol Education Program, 12, 44
LDL cholesterol and, 80, 87, 92-93, 95, 112-113, 119, 121-122, 134, 140, 162-163, 176
Niacin, 90, 94-95, 97-98, 102-103, 111, 161, 167, 169-170, 173, 176, 178-180, 182-183, 204, 208
fibrinogen and, 101-102, 173
lipoprotein (a) and, 97, 98
no-flush, 169-170
small LDL, treatment of, 94-95
Niaspan, 94-95, 173, 179, 183
small LDL, treatment of, 94-95
Nitric oxide, 160

NMR, 6, 82-83, 92, 96-97, 104-106, 173, 175, 178, 180, 239-240, *See* Nuclear magnetic resonance
  lipoproteins, 4, 6, 23, 67, 71, 73, 80-84, 87, 89, 92, 96, 102-103, 105-106, 109, 111, 126, 135, 140, 143, 153, 155, 175, 183, 185-188, 237
No-flush niacin, 169-170
Nuclear magnetic resonance, 6, 82
Nutritional supplements, 23, 88, 98, 109, 148, 155-157, 170, 187
  lipoprotein effects of, 140
Nuts, 89-90, 112, 115-116, 118, 120-121, 124-127, 129, 134, 138, 159, 163, 166, 171, 181
  LDL cholesterol and, 80, 87, 92-93, 95, 112-113, 119, 121-122, 134, 140, 162-163, 176
  monounsaturated fats and, 116, 166

O

Oat bran, 88, 95, 119-120, 124, 126-127, 162-165, 171, 174, 179
  LDL cholesterol and, 80, 87, 92-93, 95, 112-113, 119, 121-122, 134, 140, 162-163, 176
  small LDL and, 96, 109, 111, 115, 122, 126-127, 147, 153, 173
Omega-3 fatty acids, 82, 95, 114-115, 124, 157-159, 163, 166, *See* Fish oil
  flaxseed oil, 90, 114-115, 158, 164
  linolenic acid, 114, 152, 158, 163, 166
Ornish diet, 108
Ornish, MD, Dean, 24
Otvos, PhD, James, 6, 83

P

Pantetheine, 88
  LDL cholesterol and, 80, 87, 92-93, 95, 112-113, 119, 121-122, 134, 140, 162-163, 176
Pauling, PhD, Linus, 166, 167
Pecans, 120, 134, 166
Pectin, 88, 119-120
  LDL cholesterol and, 80, 87, 92-93, 95, 112-113, 119, 121-122, 134, 140, 162-163, 176
Pedometers, 153-154, 242, *See* calorie expenditure
Percentile rank, 59-61, 67, 195, 199, 201, 204
  heart attack risk and, 60-61, 198-200
Pharmax, 242
Phenylpropanolamine, 148
Phytosterols, 88, 162-164, 166, 171
  LDL cholesterol and, 80, 87, 92-93, 95, 112-113, 119, 121-122, 134, 140, 162-163, 176
Pine bark extract, 170
Plaque rupture, 8, 59, 158
Policosanol, 88, 169
  LDL cholesterol and, 80, 87, 92-93, 95, 112-113, 119, 121-122, 134, 140, 162-163, 176

Polyunsaturated fat, 115
Pravachol, 83, 93
Pravastatin, 83-84
Pregnenolone, 156
Pritikin Center, 131
Progesterone, 149-150, 155, 244
  where to obtain, 244-245
PROVE IT Trial, 83
Pseudephedrine, 148
Psyllium seed, 88, 101, 162, 164-165, 171
  LDL cholesterol and, 80, 87, 92-93, 95, 112-113, 119, 121-122, 134, 140, 162-163, 176
Pycnogenol, 170

R

Raggi, MD, Paolo, 6, 46, 60
Rath, MD, Mathias, 167
Raw nuts, 89-90, 112, 115-116, 118, 124, 126-127, 134, 163, 166, 171, 181
Red yeast, 88, 169
  LDL cholesterol and, 80, 87, 92-93, 95, 112-113, 119, 121-122, 134, 140, 162-163, 176
Reverse cholesterol transport, 81, 89, 95
Ridker, MD, Paul, 100
Rumberger, PhD, MD, John, 6, 49

S

Saturated fat, 1, 88, 110-112, 130, 152-153
Scandinavian Simvastatin Survival Study, 13
Simvastatin, 13, 80, 173, 183, 204, 208
Small LDL, 83, 89-90, 93-98, 100, 102-103, 106, 109, 111, 115, 122, 124, 126-127, 144-145,
    147, 153, 163, 165, 171, 173-181, 183
  exercise effects on, 94, 141
  fish oil and, 95, 97, 102, 183
  medical treatments, 89, 94, 143
  niacin and, 94-95
  oat bran and, 95, 127, 165, 174
Smoking, 3, 12, 16, 57, 78, 80, 110, 132, 141, 151
SourceNaturals, 241
South Beach Diet, 152
Soy protein, 88, 162, 164-165, 171, 174, 242-243
Soy protein powder, 88, 171, 174
  LDL cholesterol and, 80, 87, 92-93, 95, 112-113, 119, 121-122, 134, 140, 162-163, 176
  where to obtain, 243-244

Soyfoods Association, 243

Stanol/sterol esters, 162, *See* Phytosterols

Statin agents, 88, 91, 100, 169

   LDL cholesterol and, 80, 87, 92-93, 95, 112-113, 119, 121-122, 134, 140, 162-163, 176

Stents, 7, 16, 19, 32, 46-47, 64, 67, 79, 181

Strength training, 124, 146

stress test, 1-2, 7-8, 10, 26, 33, 36, 39, 43, 46, 48, 51, 62-64, 66, 79-80, 184, 197-198

Stress test, 1-2, 7-8, 10, 26, 33, 36, 39, 43, 46, 48, 51, 62-64, 66, 79-80, 184, 197-198

  based on heart scan score, 63, 197-98

  limitations, 30, 53, 63

Sugar-busters diet, 152

Superko, MD, Robert, 83

T

Take Control, 21, 88, 162, 171

   LDL cholesterol and, 80, 87, 92-93, 95, 112-113, 119, 121-122, 134, 140, 162-163, 176

Testosterone, 97-98, 150-152, 155-156, 174, 244

  where to obtain, 244-245

Thermogenic agents, 147-148

Tocotrienols, 167-168

Trans fatty acids, 113, 122

Triglycerides, 25, 72, 78, 82, 87, 89-92, 94, 96, 102-109, 114-115, 117, 120, 122-124, 126-127, 133, 140, 144-145, 147, 153, 157-159, 163, 165, 171, 173, 175-179, 183, 187, 201

  diet and, 1, 24, 73, 89, 101, 116, 139, 144, 149, 155, 170

  exercise effects on, 141

  fish oil and, 95, 97, 102, 183

U

Ulcerative colitis, 157, 161, 164

Ultra-fast CT, 49, 194

Ultrasound, 7, 29, 36-38, 47-48, 52-53, 159

  carotid, 18, 52-53, 159, 167

  coronary, 2-16, 18-33, 35-37, 39, 43-58, 60, 62-70, 72-73, 77-80, 82, 84, 87, 90, 92-94, 99-102, 104, 107, 109-112, 114, 126, 135, 137-139, 143, 147-148, 153, 155, 157-162, 166-168, 174, 176-178, 180-182, 185-186, 189-191, 193-209, 235, 238-239, 242

United Soybean Board, 243

V

Very low-density lipoprotein, 96

Viagra, 160

Vitamin C, 166-167, 170
Vitamin E, 167-168
VLDL, 25, 83, 89-90, 92, 96, 102, 104, 106, 109, 111, 115, 122, 124, 126-127, 144-145, 147, 153, 157-159, 171, 175, 178-179, 181, 183, *See* Very low-density lipoproteins
fish oil and, 95, 97, 102, 183

W

Walnuts, 88, 115, 120, 134, 166, 171
LDL cholesterol and, 80, 87, 92-93, 95, 112-113, 119, 121-122, 134, 140, 162-163, 176
Weight, 43, 72, 89, 93-95, 108-111, 116-118, 120, 122-123, 125-127, 133, 135, 138-141, 143-151, 153-155, 164
exercise effects on, 141, 143-147
Weight loss, 141-155
acceleration of, 143-155
calcium pyruvate and, 148
carbohydrate restriction and, 152-153
DHEA and, 151-152
diets, 89, 108-110, 112, 116, 118-119, 147, 152-153
progesterone and, 244
testosterone and, 150
Whole foods, 120-121, 135, 167, 178
Women's International Pharmacy, 244

Z

Zetia, 88, 101
C-reactive protein and, 176, 178
Zocor, 13, 80, 93, 173, 183
Zone diet, 152

0-595-31664-6

7455173R0

Made in the USA
Lexington, KY
23 November 2010